DASH DIET

100+ Tasty DASH Diet Recipes & 14-Day Food Program For Healthy Weight Loss, Effective Fat Burn, And Better Health!

TABLE OF CONTENTS

COPYRIGHT

<u>INTRODUCTION</u>

This diet, coined as the 'Healthiest Diet', is designed to provide real-life solutions to high-blood pressure by suggesting a diet that merely regulates the intake of nutrients and not alter the common diet we're all used to. Dietary Approaches to Stop Hypertension or dash focuses on controlling the intake of sodium and fats to maintain the normal blood pressure of an individual. Dash is geared towards preparing a diet that makes satisfying meals, thus, preventing people from eating in-between meals, causing loss of control over food intake. Because it keeps people from hunger in-between meals, it ideally becomes more satisfying and less controlling.

The Dash diet teaches individuals to complete the whole dash diet program by starting with stocking up the kitchen with dash-friendly food, preparing dash-friendly recipes, and performing Dash-friendly exercises. Meal plans suggested by Dash usually contain ingredients high in fibre, calcium, magnesium and potassium. Dash diets go low on sodium and sugar and emphasize the need to eat green leafy vegetables and fruits.

Avocado dip, for instance, is one of the most famous Dash diets there is today, because of its very convenient and affordable preparation. Avocado, a very rich source of monosaturated fat and lutein, (antioxidants that help protect vision), is among the many fruits that are highly-recommended for Dash diet. In this recipe, avocado has to be mashed and pitted, mixed with fat-free sour cream, onion and hot sauce. This dip shall be eaten with tortilla chips or sliced vegetables. From this dish, a person can get a total of 65 calories, 2 grams protein, 5 grams total fat, 4 grams carbohydrate, 172 milligrams potassium and 31 milligrams calcium. From this we can infer that a person is fed a considerable amount of necessary nutrients, essential for maintaining a well-balanced diet that's good for the heart.

In just 14 days, a Dash diet follower will experience normal blood pressure, with fewer tendencies to eat in-between meals, the major culprit of weight gain. The Dash diet program also teaches individuals to determine the right amount of food intake, the necessary exercise to perform according to age and activity level. Dash educates and motivates --- one of the very important reasons why people find it easy to stick to the diet. Also, the diet does not require us to give up anything significant in our usual diet, instead, it helps us create a process of adjusting to little changes so we can successfully help ourselves.

In a list of 35 popular diets for a study carried out by US News and World Report magazine the expert opinion of assembled experts gave us the verdict of The Biggest Loser diet and the DASH diet as being the best diet for diabetics, in both helping individuals to prevent the disease or for those who already have it, reversing it. But is there really a best of the best? Amongst these two champions, is there yet a champion still? I decided to do a step by step comparison in order to find out.

I compared two sample menus used by the panel assembled by and used by the US News experts. Whereas the Biggest Loser diet provided for Breakfast, snack, Lunch, Snack and dinner, the DASH diet only provided for breakfast, lunch and dinner.

A comparison of their nutritional values shows that while the Biggest Loser diet provides 1,489 calories as against the recommended daily intake of between 1600 and 2000 (depending on age) for women and between 2000 to 2400 calories (also depending on age), the DASH diet provides on its 1500 calories and 2300 calories diet 2037 and 2062 mg respectively.

An assessment of which diets calorie provision places it closest to the recommended benchmark allotted to each age grade puts the DASH diet clearly ahead of the Biggest Loser diet. As such, the first point goes to the DASH diet. For the Biggest Loser diet whilst it provides about 25 percent of your days calories, the DASH diets 26 and 27 percent respectively for its 1500 mg and 2300 mg versions. This is against the recommended daily amount of between 20 to 35 percent on these scores.

Saturated fat, both diets have down to about 5 percent, although the DASH diets 2300 mg edges further with an additional percentage (at 6 percent). These both fall within the borders of the below 10 percent recommendation. On fats therefore, I score them evenly.

Both satisfy the requirement for total carbohydrates to make up between 45 to 65 percent of daily recommended caloric intake. The Biggest Loser diet at 50 percent whilst the DASH diet at 56 and 55 percent respectively. On that note I score these diets evenly also. Both in most part equally meet the standard for fiber, although the Biggest Losers 31g falls short of the 34g recommendation for men ages 19 to 30 years old.

Further since, a fiber rich diet has been noted as a key factor in the prevention and reversal and management of diabetes, the DASH diets higher figures-36 and 37 g to the biggest Loser 31g in my opinion places the DASH diet on this score, ahead of the Biggest Loser diet.

For protein the recommended benchmark is between 10 to 35 percent of daily caloric intake. Both diets make the grade. The Biggest Loser diet at 30 percent whereas the DASH diet at the lower end of the mark at 18 percent. The reason for this latter figure pertaining to the DASH diet may be because of the avowed design of the diet to stop hypertension and thus the reduction of red meat. Nevertheless, one should note that red meat is not the only source of protein. There is white meat and protein rich legumes like beans. In addition, since a diabetic no matter which of the diet s/he is on, to make it effective, will need to complement that diet with exercise, a diet that assisting strength training through muscle health would be more advantageous. In this regard, point... goes to the Biggest Loser diet.

On Sodium or salt, the recommendation is under 2300mg and under 1500 mg for persons older than 51 years. Unfortunately, the Biggest Loser diet falls far short of this mark by being at 2904 mg clearly exceeding the limit. The DASH diet however meets it □uite well at 1507 mg for its 1500mg menu and 2101 mg for its 2300 mg menu. On that score, the point in this category is awarded it.

Next considering Potassium. The Biggest Loser diet fails to meet the recommended daily amount of at least 4700 mg. It stands at 3460 mg as against the DASH diets 4855 mg (1500 mg diet) and 4909mg (2300mg diet). Once again, the DASH diet wins the category.

With regards to Calcium intake the Biggest Loser diet performs better. Slightly edging out the DASH diets performance of 1218 mg and 120 mg for its 1500mg and 2300 mg diet versions respectively, with its own of

1128 mg. However since they both make the grade and the Biggest Losers figure is only slightly better than that for the DASH diet, they shall be awarded even scores for this category.

For vitamin B-12 too, both diets meet the mark. The Biggest Loser diet with 6.3 mg to the recommended daily amount of 2.4 mg whereas the DASH diet 4.4 mg and 6.7 mg respectively as it pertains to that diets 1500 mcg and 2300 mcg diet.

With regards to Vitamin D however, both diets apparently fail to satisfy the daily recommended amount of 15 mcg. Thus whilst the DASH diet comes in at 11 mcg, the Biggest Loser diet edges it ever so slightly at 11.4mcg. However this is not enough for us to award the Biggest Loser diet a win for this category, especially since it did not meet the recommended daily amount.

As concerns recommended daily amounts, it should be noted that this appellation applies to adults 19 years and over and that it assumes them a sedentary lifestyle.

Nevertheless, the results are now all in. Having it that the DASH diet bests the Biggest Loser diet in the categories recommended daily caloric intake, provisions for fiber, sodium and potassium and the BIGGEST Loser diet only winning in the protein category and both being awarded even scores in the rest, it can clearly be seen that the DASH diet has carried the day. Furthermore, it can honestly be said to be not only the best diabetes diet but all things considered, premised on studies made and the fact that it was actually designed to help stop hypertension, it may just be for now, the best general purpose diet out there.

However having said this, it cannot be over-emphasized that diabetics and others should take care to consult their doctors first before embarking on any diet regimen or exercise.

Importance Of Dash Diet

High blood pressure, or hypertension, can increase the risk of heart attack, heart failure, stroke, and kidney disease.

Experts who reviewed the DASH diet in 2017, 20 years after its launch, described it as an intervention that could considerably boost the health of the population. According to the review, if people with high blood pressure followed the DASH diet precisely, this could prevent around 400,000 deaths from cardiovascular disease over 10 years.

Who can benefit?

According to an article from 2019, people who follow the DASH diet can reduce levels of:

- ✓ blood pressure
- ✓ blood sugar
- ✓ triglycerides, or fat, in the blood
- ✓ low-density lipoprotein (LDL), or "bad" cholesterol

insulin resistance

These are all features of metabolic syndrome, a condition that also involves obesity, type 2 diabetes, and a higher risk of cardiovascular disease. A 2013 study looked at the impact of DASH on people with and without metabolic syndrome who followed the diet for 8 weeks.

Results showed that on average:

- In people with metabolic syndrome, the systolic pressure fell by 4.9 millimeters of mercury (mm Hg), and the diastolic fell by 1.9 mm HG.

- In people without metabolic syndrome, the systolic pressure fell by 5.2 mm Hg, and the diastolic fell by 2.9 mm Hg.

In other words, DASH can be effective at lowering blood pressure in people with or without metabolic syndrome. There is also evidence that it may reduce the risk of colorectal cancer and improve overall life expectancy.

The National Kidney Foundation recommend DASH for people with kidney disease.

There are two versions of the DASH diet:

1. The Standard DASH diet: People consume up to 2,300 milligrams (mg) of sodium each day.

2. The Low Sodium DASH diet: The maximum sodium intake is 1,500 mg each day.

Many people in the U.S. consume 3,600 mg of sodium or more each day, so both versions of the DASH diet aim to reduce sodium consumption.

In a clinical trial to assess the diet's impact, experts found that combining the DASH diet with a low sodium intake has more impact on blood pressure than taking just one of these actions.

As people reduce their salt intake, they should also eat more foods that contain potassium. Potassium helps the blood vessels relax, and this can lower blood pressure. People should aim to consume 4,700 mg of potassium each day.

Foods that contain potassium include:

- ✓ dried fruit, such as apricots, prunes, and raisins
- ✓ lentils and kidney beans
- ✓ s□uash
- ✓ potato
- ✓ orange juice
- ✓ banana

A half-cup of dried apricots will provide around 30% of a person's daily need for potassium. A cup of cooked lentils provides 21%. The Mediterranean diet may also benefit the heart and overall health.

CHAPTER ONE

HOW DOES DASH DIET WORKS

Perhaps you have heard of the DASH Diet for Hypertension. Well, it is actually among the most renowned diet plans out there nowadays and it may be more than a trend. Designed by the US Department of Health and Human Services' National Institutes of Health, this diet program is founded on nutritional facts.

DASH is an acronym for Dietary Approaches to Stop Hypertension, this basically means, tips on how to decrease your blood pressure levels via the foods you ingest. The premise of the diet plan is to guide men and women with high blood pressure and hypertension on out how to eat much healthier and reduce their blood pressure and the possibility of connected ailments. High blood pressure is often a problem that might be easily avoided by leading a healthy life-style nevertheless, once a person has it, it can only be managed.

Having elevated blood pressure is a serious matter and may even bring about illnesses such as coronary artery disease, dementia, stroke and eventually heart failure. Picture this, close to 33% of men and women currently have high blood pressure or hypertension. That's one third of the adult populace, and therefore there exists a very good probability that either you or somebody you know may possibly be identified as having the ailment.

The DASH Diet for Hypertension may help you reduce your blood pressure and also your potential risk for some of the affiliated ailments through setting a few rules to go by. To illustrate, one of the main recommendations set forth by the weight loss plan is to reduce your sodium consumption to between 2,300 and 1,500 mg a day. This may look like you are still receiving a large amount of sodium, but in reality it is not very much. Consider some of the items you might consume every single day.

Were you aware that a quarter pounder with cheese provides approximately 1,190 milligrams of sodium? That's basically your entire daily allowance if you are limiting yourself to 1,500 milligrams a day. Even at 2,300 per day, it is still over 50 percent the suggested daily portion. Even if you imagine you are going to be health conscious and get salad, be warned. Condiments and dressings have proven to be notorious for including large levels of sodium.

So, what will you end up taking in on The DASH Diet?

- Plenty of vegetables and fruits per day in place of sweets and desserts
- Foods which are high in dietary fiber as an alternative to refined carbs
- Low-fat and fat-free dairy products rather than whole milk products
- Water and club soda as opposed to sugary soft drinks

The DASH Diet is not just an agenda pertaining to eating, it advises some healthy lifestyle changes as well:

- Initiate a workout plan whether or not your blood pressure level is typical
- Try to get at least thirty minutes of physical exercise on a daily basis
- Determine weight reduction targets for yourself

If you take prescription medication for high blood pressure, don't forget to take it daily

With such common sense advice it's no surprise The DASH Diet is gaining this sort of interest at this moment. This is a diet plan that makes sense and offers the potential to enable you to lose weight and remain healthful. Even people who have healthy blood pressure can usually benefit from the DASH Diet and sticking to a high fiber, low fat, minimal sodium eating routine. Pursuing this diet will not just allow you to shed pounds, it could actually help save your life.

3 Phase Liver Detox Diet Cleansing - How Does It Work?

You must have learnt in your biology classes about the importance of the liver. Your liver is the largest internal organ in your body and it performs well over 500 chemical functions. One of the most important functions of liver is it filters out the toxins and the chemicals that enter your body and stops them from going into your blood. Over time your liver becomes sluggish because of accumulated toxins. It is important to remove the toxic accumulation from the liver and this is why a liver detox is important. There are several ways of detoxifying the liver - one of the best ways is liver detox diet.

Preparing It

Before starting with liver detox diet you will need to plan out everything carefully. Planning is important because you need to prepare your body for the diet. Preparing the body will give you maximum benefits of the detox program. Now the big question is how will you prepare? The first thing that you will need to do is stay away from caffeine, alcohol, junk food, decaf and meat. Before you start with the detox diet eat only vegetables and fruits for a week. Cut down on your sugar intake and increase the intake of water and whole wheat bread. Carry on with the detox diet in three phases over a period of one week.

First Phase

The first phase of the detox diet will span from the first to the third day. You will have to survive solely on liquid. Have 10-12 glasses of water with a dash of lemon juice daily. This will help in detoxification and will flush out the accumulated wastes. Stay away from other beverages and dairy products. This will relax your liver and the digestive system. You may experience a bit of tiredness - don't worry. It happens because all the wastes are being flushed out of your system. During this phase you can have rosemary tea if you want to.

Second Phase

The second phase of the liver detoxification diet will continue for the next three days. You can include fruits, vegetables and semi solid food in your diet during this phase. Opt for vegetables and fruits that are organically grown. You need to continue drinking 12 glasses of water in this phase too. Fresh fruit juices are great for liver detox. So each morning prepare of orange, apple, celery or carrot juice. Every evening have a vegetable broth made with carrots, spinach potato and broccoli. In this phase too, you can continue having the rosemary tea.

Third Phase

The third phase of the liver detoxification diet will last only for the seventh day. Include 12 glasses of water, rosemary tea, fresh fruit and organically grown vegetables in your diet. Raw vegetables are good for liver detoxification. However you can steam your vegetables if you want to. To conclude the diet program successfully go back to your normal diet gradually. Stay away from alcohol for at least a week after the diet program ends.

Food To Eat And Avoid On Dash Diet

Before we get into specific foods, you should familiarize yourself with the DASH diet food serving guidelines. The DASH eating plan dictates a certain number of daily servings from food groups. For instance, in a 2,000-calorie diet, a person would include:

- ✓ Whole grains: 6-8 servings per day
- ✓ Vegetables: 4-5 servings per day
- ✓ Fruits: 4-5 servings per day
- ✓ Fat-free or low-fat milk and milk products: 2-3 servings per day
- ✓ Lean meat, poultry, and fish: 6 ounces or less per day
- ✓ Nuts, seeds, and legumes: 4-5 servings per week
- ✓ Fats and oils: 2-3 servings per day
- ✓ Sweets and added sugars: 5 servings or less per week
- ✓ Maximum sodium limit: 2,300 milligrams per day or 1,500 milligrams per day

Before we get into exactly which foods are included in these food groups, we'll discuss which foods the DASH diet recommends you cut from your diet.

What foods you should avoid on the DASH diet.

The DASH diet limits foods that will negatively impact your blood pressure and heart health. The following foods should be avoided when following the eating plan.

1. High-sodium foods

Studies have shown that drastically cutting back on dietary salt is associated with decreased risk of hypertension, heart disease, and stroke. Not sprinkling salt on your meals is one of the biggest challenges followers of the DASH diet face. However, salt reduction is integral to the plan, so opt for herbs and spices instead.

- Table salt
- Fast food
- Pre-packaged food
- Processed meats

Red meats

According to a 1999 study, the DASH diet emphasizes fish and chicken over red meat. Though it's not strictly forbidden, red meat consumption should be limited since it's high in saturated fat and cholesterol.

- ✓ Beef
- ✓ Pork
- ✓ Lamb
- ✓ Veal

Saturated fat

There's conflicting reports whether saturated fat is linked to heart disease. The DASH diet plays it safe and recommends reducing your intake of foods high in saturated fat.

- ✓ Cheese
- ✓ Fatty cuts of meat
- ✓ Poultry with skin
- ✓ Lard
- ✓ Cream
- ✓ Butter
- ✓ Whole milk

Added sugar

If you follow the DASH diet, you'll want to get used to reading ingredient labels on packaged foods and skip out on adding sugar cubes to your tea. Although research on sugar and hypertension is limited, some evidence supports that sugar may increase blood pressure. There may not be a conclusive link between the two, but it's still a good idea to cut back on added sugar; sugar is high in calories and yet adds no nutritional value.

- ✓ Table sugar
- ✓ Sweets
- ✓ Condiments with added sugar
- ✓ Junk food

What foods can you eat on the DASH diet?

Now that we've got what you should cut back on out of the way, now it's time to learn about which DASH diet foods you can happily eat more of.

Whole grains

Servings: 6-8 per day

With a recommended 6 to 8 servings a day, whole grains are the foundation of the DASH diet for their ability to reduce the risk of hypertension. While this may seem like a lot, it's as simple as having whole grain cereal or oatmeal for breakfast and quinoa, brown rice, or wheat pasta with lunch and dinner.

- ✓ Whole-wheat bread
- ✓ Whole-wheat pasta
- ✓ Oatmeal
- ✓ Brown rice
- ✓ Unsalted pretzels
- ✓ Popcorn

Fruits

Servings: 4 to 5 servings per day

All fruits are compliant on the DASH diet. In fact, the diet encourages eating them. Let go of your fear that the natural sugar in fruit is bad for you. Enjoy 4 to 5 servings per day in the form of snacks, smoothies, toppings, and dessert. Limit serving sizes to 1/2 cup fresh fruit and 1/4 cup for dried fruit.

- ✓ Apples
- ✓ Bananas
- ✓ Dates
- ✓ Grapes
- ✓ Oranges
- ✓ Peaches
- ✓ Raisins
- ✓ Strawberries

Vegetables

Servings: 5 to 6 servings per day

Everyone's favorite food group: Vegetables. As you get older, veggies become less scary. On this diet, you'll want to pack in 5 to 6 servings daily. Try making soups, salads, and side dishes with old favorites like peas and carrots and don't be afraid to try new vegetables like spaghetti squash.

- ✓ Broccoli
- ✓ Carrots
- ✓ Collards
- ✓ Green peas
- ✓ Potatoes
- ✓ Spinach

Lean proteins

Servings: 6 ounces per day

The DASH diet was inspired by the vegetarian lifestyle, but this diet isn't all plant-based. You can eat a maximum of 6 ounces of lean meat or eggs per day. This doesn't seem like a lot, but less meat may be better for patients with hypertension and heart health risks anyway. Stick with poultry and fish, and avoid frying. Vegans and vegetarians can opt for tofu and tempeh.

- ✓ Broiled, roasted, or poached meat
- ✓ Skinless chicken
- ✓ Eggs
- ✓ Fish

Low-Fat Dairy

Servings: 2-3 per day

The diet recommends avoiding high levels of saturated fat, so swap out your whole dairy products for low-fat or fat-free. You can still enjoy 2 to 3 servings of dairy products per day as long as they're low in fat and sodium.

- ✓ Fat-free milk

✓ Low-fat cheese

✓ Fat-free or low-fat yogurt

Nuts, seeds, and legumes

Servings: 4-5 per week

The DASH Diet recommends consuming this food group 4 to 5 times per week. Nuts and seeds are excellent sources of healthy fats while legumes, such as beans and lentils, are good sources of plant protein and rich in fiber. The DASH diet emphasizes increasing fiber intake, and these high fiber foods will help you do that. These are all sources of many vital vitamins and minerals, too. The servings are fewer than the other food groups, however, and this is because these foods tend to be higher in calories.

✓ Almonds

✓ Walnuts

✓ Sunflower seeds

✓ Peanut butter

✓ Kidney beans

✓ Lentils

✓ Split peas

Heart-healthy oils

Servings: 2 to 3 servings per day

Aspects of the DASH diet are inspired by the Mediterranean diet, which is high in healthy fats. Heart-healthy fats are an important part of the DASH diet, too, which is why followers consume 2 to 3 servings per day of monounsaturated fats. Your go-to oil will probably be olive oil.

- ✓ Olive oil
- ✓ Canola oil
- ✓ Safflower oil
- ✓ Low-fat mayonnaise

Low fat sweets

Servings: 5 or less per week

You're better off without sugar, though the creators of the DASH diet understand that you'll want to treat yourself occasionally. In that case, they've recommended some approved sugars you can indulge in 5 or less times per week.

The DASH diet-approved sweets are all low in fat and include:

- ✓ Fruit-flavored gelatin

- ✓ Jelly
- ✓ Maple syrup
- ✓ Sorbet and ices

What foods and drinks should be avoided while following a DASH diet?

Foods and drinks to avoid when following the DASH diet include high sugar, high fat snacks, and foods high in salt such as:

- Candy
- Cookies
- Chips
- Salted nuts
- Sodas
- Sugary beverages
- Pastries
- Snacks
- Meat dishes

Prepackaged pasta and rice dishes (excluding macaroni and cheese because it is a separate category)

- Pizza
- Soups

- Salad dressings

- Cheese

- Cold cuts and cured meats

- Breads and rolls

- Sandwiches

- Sauces and gravies

- Soups

Using a salt substitute made with potassium not only works as a substitute in cooking and on the table, but the additional potassium can help lower blood pressure. People who are on blood pressure medications that increase potassium should ask their doctors to help them monitor the blood level of potassium (K) while they are making changes.

What about red meat and heart disease?

While not specifically recommended, grass-fed beef and buffalo would fit within these parameters. Grass-fed beef has a very different composition than conventional grain-fed beef. Grass-fed beef is high in omega-3s and is more similar to fish, nutritionally. Grain-fed red meat is high in omega 6s and saturated fat, both of which are promote inflammation and contribute to heart disease, high blood pressure, and obesity. Red meat that is not grass-fed is not allowed.

Putting the pieces of the DASH diet together

Try these strategies to get started on the DASH diet:

> **Change gradually.**

If you now eat only one or two servings of fruits or vegetables a day, try to add a serving at lunch and one at dinner. Rather than switching to all whole grains, start by making one or two of your grain servings whole grains. Increasing fruits, vegetables and whole grains gradually can also help prevent bloating or diarrhea that may occur if you aren't used to eating a diet with lots of fiber. You can also try over-the-counter products to help reduce gas from beans and vegetables.

> **Reward successes and forgive slip-ups.**

Reward yourself with a nonfood treat for your accomplishments — rent a movie, purchase a book or get together with a friend. Everyone slips, especially when learning something new. Remember that changing your lifestyle is a long-term process. Find out what triggered your setback and then just pick up where you left off with the DASH diet.

> ➢ **Add physical activity.**

To boost your blood pressure lowering efforts even more, consider increasing your physical activity in addition to following the DASH diet. Combining both the DASH diet and physical activity makes it more likely that you'll reduce your blood pressure.

Get support if you need it. If you're having trouble sticking to your diet, talk to your doctor or dietitian about it. You might get some tips that will help you stick to the DASH diet.

Remember, healthy eating isn't an all-or-nothing proposition. What's most important is that, on average, you eat healthier foods with plenty of variety — both to keep your diet nutritious and to avoid boredom or extremes. And with the DASH diet, you can have both.

DASH Diet to Solve Hypertension

DASH stands for Dietary Approaches for Stopping Hypertension. It is a common term used by physicians all over the United States. Basically it involves a diet which consists of foods that have proven to lower high blood pressure, or hypertension. Of course, the DASH diet also calls for a minimization of foods that are well known to contribute to high blood pressure as well.

The DASH diet is not truly defined by any means, and therefore is broad in its various executions. However, the guidelines that the DASH diet gives to people with hypertension have shown to enable them to lower their blood pressure in a matter of weeks, with drastic improvements for periods over six months of DASH dieting. This drastic improvement has led to its increased and continued usage of the DASH diet by physicians across the country.

The components of the DASH diet are very simple, and are easy to follow. The major contributors to the lowering of participants' blood pressure are the fruits, vegetables, legumes, seeds, and nuts. The good cholesterol, fiber, and negative calories are all good components of a well balanced and healthy diet. Olive oil is also encouraged, and has shown to contribute lower blood pressures with studies throughout the Mediterranean countries and their inhabitants which use olive oil daily.

Another healthy change that the DASH diet brings to the average American diet are the low-fat items. For instance, the DASH diet recommends low-fat dairy products and lean meats such as poultry and fish. Now, some fish contain more fats than others, so it is important for you to balance your intake between the two. Besides, the fattier fishes are actually more expensive on average! Finally, it is important for you to take in several whole grain products each day. Oatmeal for breakfast is a popular solution, as well as granola bars as between-meal snacks.

The most important step in the DASH diet is to minimize foods and items which contribute to high blood pressure. The main contributors to hypertension are inactivity, excess sodium, excess alcohol, excess body weight, and inade□uate magnesium, potassium, and calcium. If you also noticed, DASH diet foods are also foods that are recommended for weight loss diets. The reason that these foods are found in the DASH diet and in weight loss diets is due to the fact that most people with hypertension are usually overweight. The most effective treatment for hypertension, disclosed by most physicians, is weight loss.

One of the closest diets that you can compare to the DASH diet is the Vegan diet. I was able to write an article recently, "Make The Vegetarian Diet Work For You", which explains the benefits and uses of Vegan foods towards your health. A lot of the foods that you see recommended in the DASH diet are also foods that are a part of the Vegan diet, which would explain the fact that Vegan's are very rarely diagnosed with hypertension.

Proper documentation on the DASH diet is available from your physician, as well as at several online dietary sources. I would definitely recommend researching DASH diet foods and to start planning your daily diet around them immediately. The health benefits that you will see with the lowered blood pressure is important in the short term for better health and well-being, however it is critical in the long term. The DASH diet will help to extend your life due to your cardiovascular system's inability to operate for years under a higher pressure than what it is designed for. You also will be able to access dietary tips and extensive information at my website listed below. My free membership fitness tuning site focuses on dietary as well as fitness aspects in order to contribute towards a healthy lifestyle for people of all ages and body types.

High Blood Pressure and The DASH Diet

High blood pressure or hypertension is a primary risk factor for conditions such as stroke, heart attack and kidney damage. Your blood pressure (BP) is taken using a sphygmomanometer and is a measurement of the force re□uired for your heart to pump blood through the arteries to the organs and tissues in your body. It is divided into what is called the systolic pressure and the diastolic pressure. The systolic pressure is the top number, while the diastolic pressure is the bottom number. The systolic measurement is recorded when the heart contracts, and should be around 120 millimeters of mercury (mmHg) in a healthy adult, while the diastolic measurement is recorded as the heart relaxes and is usually around 80 millimeters of mercury (mmHg) in a healthy adult. You'll see this blood pressure reading written down as 120/80.

In Australia, there are around three million adults with high blood pressure. The main problem with this condition is that you don't feel it, so it can be present without diagnosis for many years, until it causes a serious medical emergency such as a heart attack or stroke. In the past, hypertension was considered to be a condition of 'old age'. However, the current research suggests that high blood pressure can be prevented if we lead a healthy lifestyle, by eating a well balanced diet that reduces excess sugar and saturated fat, increases the level of fibre, as well as vitamins, minerals and antioxidants. Following a regular exercise or physical activity program also helps to keep the heart healthy by making the muscles more efficient at utilizing oxygen and other nutrients from the blood.

Some people have a genetic predisposition, making them more likely to develop it if they had a parent who had hypertension, or suffered from a heart attack or stroke in their middle age. Your chances of developing high blood pressure will be increased by one or more of the following issues:

✓ Excess abdominal fat
✓ High alcohol consumption
✓ High salt intake
✓ High sugar and refined carbohydrate intake
✓ Chronic stress

- ✓ Lack of physical activity
- ✓ Sedentary job

One dietary approach that is backed up by □uality research is the DASH (Dietary Approaches to Stop Hypertension) Diet. This dietary approach includes lean meat, chicken and fish (rich in omega-3 fats) with fresh fruits and vegetables, low-fat dairy foods, nuts and whole grains. This diet is low in saturated fat and recommends eliminating excess sugar from sweets, sugary drinks and other forms of junk food. In 1997, the New England Journal of Medicine published the earliest results showing success using the DASH Diet. Since these first clinical results were published, many other clinical studies have confirmed the effectiveness of using the DASH Diet as a way of reducing blood pressure.

CHAPTER TWO

DIET MINDSET

Dieting has long been used as a method for people to lose weight. However the truth is that not only does dieting guarantee your failure, but it may also be the □uickest way to gain weight. Yes, dieting actually makes you fat! It is commonly used because initially you will lose weight, but then when the "backlash" occurs you will gain it all back and then some. The reason dieting it is so effective at making you fat is that it changes you in 3 fundamental ways - physiologically, psychologically, and neurologically.

Being able to understand those 3 big words isn't important, what is important is how they affect you and your weight. Each re□uire their own separate article, and in this one, I am going to discuss how dieting changes you psychologically. Psychology has no formal definition, so to make matters easy to understand we are going to talk of psychology as "the way you think". This article will therfore outline some ways in which dieting makes you fat simply by altering the way that you think.

1. "All or Nothing" Thinking:

All or nothing thinking is when you are either ON your diet, or you are OFF your diet. People who have this thinking usually do quite well when they are "on" their diet. They remain disciplined and focused on their objective of losing weight. It's when they are "off" their diet that chaos occurs. It's a Dr.Jekyll vs Mr.Hyde scenario. As soon as Dr.Jekyll breaks loose, all or nothing thinkers break into a frenzy - late night binges, ice-cream gorges, all you can eat buffets, and anything else you can think of. Here is what goes through the mind of an "all or nothing" thinker:

"I'm off my diet so I am going to eat whatever I want and I can always go back on a diet if I need to but I don't even care because I just want to eat this delicious food. I'll just start my new diet on Monday and no matter what I am going to stick to that diet."

2. "Get it all in" Thinking:

"Get it all in" thinking is really popular among long term dieters. "Get it all on" thinking occurs between the period when you decide you are going on a diet and when you actually start. Here is what goes through the mind of a "get it all in" thinker:

"I have to eat absolutely everything that I love and stuff myself full, because as soon as I go on my diet I will never be able to eat these foods again so I need to eat as much as I can now because the is the last time I will ever eat these foods."

3. "I can go on a diet" Thinking:

Again this one is very common among chronic dieters. It's most common among people who do quite well on diets initially, those who lose around 10-15 pounds before they relapse and gain the weight back. Dieters who have this thinking know that if they want to lose weight they can simply go on a diet whenever they want, and so they use that excuse to eat whatever they want. Their thinking goes something like this:

"It doesn't matter if I eat all this now because I can always go on a diet tomorrow if I want to. In fact I should just eat what I want for the next week because I will only gain a few pounds at most and that doesn't really matter because I can lose it easily anyway"

4. "I broke my diet" Thinking:

"I broke my diet" thinking happens when you are on a specific diet and you end up eating something that you were not supposed to. Then because you just "broke" your diet you decide to eat whatever you want and to start again another time. "I broke my diet" thinking goes something like this:

"Oh my god I just broke my diet I can't believe how much of a slob I am, I am so useless I can't even stick to a simple diet. Well now that I have broken it I may as well eat whatever I want because it doesn't even matter anymore. I guess I will just eat everything and start again on Monday."

Those are just a few of the ways in which dieting can change the way that you think about food and your weight. If you are trying to lose weight by dieting then it is common that you will have experienced at least one or maybe all of these ways of thinking. It's not your fault, these psychological "tricks" are hard-wired into our brains because we were never supposed to consciously restrict ourselves from food.

Dieting is a behavior that will give you short term results, but your body and brain will find ways to reverse that in the long run. Unless your goal is to actually gain weight, dieting is a terrible solution to any problem. It's simply not good for you, and it is an activity that can never be maintained.

Ways to Shift Your Mindset for Better Weight Loss

"Shifting your mindset about how to lose weight is the biggest factor in losing weight," "We can't shift our weight from the outside without realizing the correct inner resolve and intention."

And most people try to lose weight with the worst state of mind possible: wanting to "fix" themselves. They jump into diets and exercise plans out of self-deprecation, all the while pinching their "trouble" spots, calling themselves "fat" and feeling altogether less-than. They get obsessed with results, focus on uick fixes and lose sight of sustainability and even health.

"This type of thinking can be destructive," says board-certified North Carolina internal medicine physician Dr. Kevin Campbell. "Rather than focusing on the good that can come of weight loss – such as better health, a longer life, more enjoyment in everyday activities and the prevention of diabetes and heart disease – these folks focus on negative thoughts. Ultimately, a negative mindset leads to failure."

Yes, shifting your attitude around weight loss isn't just about feel-goodery; it's about results. In fact, research from Syracuse University shows that the more dissatisfied women are with their bodies, the more likely they are to avoid exercise. And simply thinking that you're overweight predicts future weight gain.

While psychologists stress that how you see yourself and your core identity predicts your actions (see yourself as overweight, averse to exercise or unworthy, and you'll act accordingly), biology may also play a role. Research published in Psychosomatic Medicine even show that the stress hormone cortisol, which your adrenal glands secrete every time you get down on yourself or worry about how you measure up on the scale, increases distribution of fat around the abdomen.

Fortunately, the mind is a flexible thing. Follow these 10 expert-approved tips to change your mindset and make your weight-loss approach healthier, happier and way more effective:

1. Change Your Goals

Losing weight might be a result, but it shouldn't be the goal. Rather, your goals should small, sustainable things over which you have full control, says NYC-based therapist Paul Hokemeyer. Did you eat five servings of fruits and veggies today? There's one goal met. What about eight hours of sleep; did you get them in? If so, you can check another goal off of your list.

2. Gravitate to Positivity

"Surround yourself with positive people," Smerling says. Doing so provides you an encouraging, emotionally healthy environment in which to invest in yourself. "Don't be afraid to ask for help or support," says Chicago-based Nike NTC master trainer and run coach Emily Hutchins.

3. Rethink Rewards and Punishments

"Keep in mind that making healthy choices is a way of practicing self-care,"." Food is not a reward, and exercise is not a punishment. They are both ways of caring for your body and helping you feel your best. You deserve both.

4. Take a Breath

Taking a few minutes at the beginning of your workout, or even at the beginning of your day, to slow down and simply focus on the act of breathing can help you set your intentions, connect with your body and even lower your body's stress response, Hutchins says. Lie on your back with your legs extended and place one hand on your stomach and one on your chest. Breathe in through your nose for four seconds, hold for two and then exhale through your mouth for six. With each breath, the hand placed on your stomach should be the only one to rise or fall.

5. Throw Out the Calendar

"Patience is also important when you are losing weight in a healthy and sustainable matter," Plus, if you focus on meeting truly actionable goals, like taking 10,000 steps each and every day, there's no need to get wrapped up in a timeline of goals ahead. Every 24 hours comes with new successes; focus on those.

6. Identify Your 'Trouble Thoughts'

"Identify the thoughts that get you into trouble and work to stop and change them. Maybe it's your internal dialogue when you look into the mirror. Or cravings when you get stressed. "Consciously make them stop by saying 'stop' out loud," she says. It might sound silly, but that simple action will break your chain of thought and allow yourself the opportunity to introduce a new, healthier one. "The best way to do this is to count from one to 100 as many times as you need until the destructive thoughts subside.

7. Don't Step on the Scale

While the scale isn't intrinsically bad, a lot of us have learned to associate it with self-destructive thoughts and actions. If that's you, don't even bother stepping on the scale until you get to a place in which the number on the scale doesn't define your worth,

8. Talk to Yourself Like You Would a Friend

"When it comes to ideals of beauty and body image, we are incredibly hard on ourselves. The standards we adopt for ourselves are punishing. And we'd never hold our friends or loved ones to many of those standards. You deserve the same respect and compassion as anyone else; treat yourself like it.

9. Forget the Whole 'Foods Are Good or Bad' Mentality

Somewhere along the line, we've learned to feel either proud or guilty about every food choice we make. But it's just food, and you shouldn't have to feel guilty about wanting the occasional cookie. "Give yourself permission to have a glass wine or a piece of chocolate cake. "Remember, all foods fit."

10. Focus on the Attainable

"If you have never stepped into a gym before, your goal shouldn't be doing 30 minutes on the elliptical on day one. A better goal may be to go for a 20-minute walk," she says. "If you want to cook more, but have little experience with healthy recipes or are strapped for time, don't expect yourself to craft new healthy recipes every night after work. Maybe consider using a delivery service such as HelloFresh or Blue Apron in which pre-portioned ingredients and recipes are sent to your door, helping you to get acquainted with new ingredients, try out new recipes and build fundamental cooking skills." Start where you are and build from there.

CHAPTER THREE

THE SECRET OF DASH DIET FOOD

Be wary of fad diet trends. Good reasons exist to restrict certain types of foods from your diet, but in many cases, people flock to fad diet trends as a way to lose weight, not because of a particular medical condition. The biggest drawback to fad diets: they don't alter long-term eating behavior and are not sustainable for a lifetime.

If you're looking for an easy to follow, evidence-based diet that you can stay on forever, The DASH Diet could your ticket to better health. The secret? It's proven. Due to its namesake, Dietary Approaches to Stop Hypertension, the research for this diet began as an approach to lower blood pressure. But what's really cool is that after several research trials, it was also recognized to support weight loss, diabetes control, and even bone health.

Eating the DASH way is sustainable too (as in, you can keep it up long-term) – something that many fad diets can't brag about. We all want instant gratification sometimes, but eating well is something that we have to do for a lifetime. Focus on adding foods to your diet, like a variety of fresh fruits and vegetables, fat-free or low-fat milk products, whole grains and lean meats, instead of taking away!

Easy Tips for Starting DASH Today:

1. Add fruit, protein and fiber to your breakfast. Add sliced banana or blueberries to your oatmeal. Top with a tablespoon of chopped nuts.

2. Enjoy 4-8 ounces of yogurt for a mid-morning or mid-day snack

3. At lunchtime, add protein to a salad – try 3-4 ounces grilled salmon or chicken on a bed of mixed greens with a vinaigrette dressing. Or top salad greens with dried cranberries, 1 tablespoon sunflower seeds, and cottage cheese.

4. Prepare extra veggies ahead. Steam, grill, or sauté a larger amount of your favorite vegetable (spinach, zucchini, broccoli, peppers, onions, or green beans). Use over the next 2-3 days for lunch or dinners, or to mix into a grain dish.

5. Take a good look at your plate. Balance your plate with half fruits/vegetables, a smaller

portion of protein, and a small portion of high fiber grain.

Exercise coupled with a nutritious diet plan is a great way to lose weight. Starving yourself to death and doing nothing is not an effective method of losing those unwanted love handles. You can even get sick if you do not do it properly.

Our body needs food, whether we like it or not. Like car parts, our major organs might not work properly if not given fuel (food). If we stop eating right, we start losing oxygen in our bloodstreams and this can create certain problems in regards to our health. In order to keep healthy we need to eat the right nutritious food that our body needs.

There are a lot of people who discovered the benefits of drinking vegetable juice. It is said that certain vegetables can help fight illnesses and even cancer. These people are not only getting healthy but they have started losing weight.

Vegetable juice is great due to its calorie content. A glassful of vegetable juice only has 46 calories on it. it is packed with vitamins and nutrients that can keep you living healthier and longer. But it is advisable that you make your own veggie juice at home. Commercial vegetable juice has a lot of sodium content added to it during processing. To avoid this you can just purchase an electric juicer and enjoy your juice daily, right in the comfort of your own home.

Another good thing about vegetable juice is that you will not have to take time to slice, dice, or cook it before you can enjoy your meal. With a juicer you can just put a whole carrot, or even add some parsley to it, and then you can drink it up. You can even add some spices like cayenne pepper, cardamom, or allspice. You might think this funny but adding a dash of spice in your veggie juice can boost your metabolism and help you lose weight fast.

Some people try juicing for 5 whole days in a month. This can help them lose weight through a detoxification process. This eliminates and melts those unwanted fats away. But before dieting, just for precautionary measures, it is wise to first ask your doctor about it.

Break the Dieting Routine

Instead of focusing on the latest fad diet, it's really as simple as eating the foods that are going to take extra weight off and keep you trim, and that will help fight chronic diseases like diabetes, heart disease and even cancer.

You can incorporate all the healthful foods you can imagine into a diet abundant in flavor, satisfaction and vibrance without having to even think about your waist line again. To many people this concept seems so easy that they think it's a gimmick, until they give it a try.

Sure, this means cutting out things like fast food and soda. But in the long run you won't even want anything to do with these foods anymore! However, there are numerous foods you can enjoy that will easily take the place of fast foods and sugary drinks. For example you can have homemade chili cheese nachos or pizza for dinner anytime you want without gaining weight, as long as you make it yourself and you use the right ingredients.

What are The Right Ingredients?

The right things to use when preparing foods for weight loss and for healthy living are those that don't come in a can or a box. Instead of buying it canned, make your own chili from scratch using a mixture of pinto and black beans and adding dice tomatoes, chili peppers, bell peppers, corn, chili powder and a dash of cumin.

Instead of purchasing frozen or pre-cooked French fries, cut up your own potatoes into wedges, toss them in olive oil and a little salt, and roast them in the oven. Another easy way to spruce up a not so healthy food is to replace white pasta with whole wheat versions, and to use brown or wild rice.

Here are some of the things you can do to get rid of your negative mindset:

1. Turn your bad habits into good:

I know this is tough, but not impossible. Do you always eat more than you should? Studies point out that most people overeat not out of hunger but for the purpose of deriving emotional comfort from foods! Since no other food could give anyone more pleasure and comfort than junk foods, so these people gorge on them as much as they can! Unless you can get rid of this unhealthy eating habit, you cannot expect to lose weight!

The first step to get rid of this habit is to realize that food cannot comfort you in any way; if you are depressed, frustrated, or simply bored, you need to find other ways to change the negativity of your life into something positive. For example, if you are bored on Sunday because you have nothing to do, why don't you go for swimming, or basketball, or any other activity you like?

If you keep yourself busy in various different activities, you won't even know when and how your time has passed! And what is more - you won't feel any need to eat junk foods! Plus, if you keep yourself active, you will also be able to lose weight and stay fit. Talk about killing two birds with one stone!

2. Think like a winner:

Stop thinking like a loser all the time and start thinking like a winner! Believe it or not, you can achieve what you want, if only you change your mindset and attitude! One thing you can do is to make two lists: one detailing your various strengths and talents, and another about the obstacles and barriers that are keeping you from succeeding in your weight loss goals!

CHAPTER FOUR

DASH DIET AND DISEASE

In the last 50 years in the United States, clinicians have seen a rise in diseases including hypertension (HTN), diabetes, obesity, and coronary artery disease (CAD). An estimated 2000 people die of heart disease every day in the United States. Chronic diseases related to diet and obesity have become major causes of death in the United States across all ethnicities. Obesity has been linked to the major etiological factor in diabetes, HTN, cancer, and CAD.

Although there have been several advancements in the scientific world regarding new medications and cutting-edge diagnostic techniques, the rate of these diseases has multiplied many times. This increase has been steep particularly in the last 20 years. Due to this trend, major organizations including the American Heart Association, National Institutes of Health, and National Heart, Lung, and Blood Institute have all started looking at an integrative approach to managing this growing epidemic. Diagnostic testing and medications are still the mainstays of patient management. However, the importance of diet, exercise, stress reduction, and lifestyle habits cannot be ignored.

A typical modern North American diet is high in saturated fats, omega-6 fatty acids, high glycemic load carbohydrates, and many artificial additives. This unhealthy diet, combined with little training in nutrition among medical professionals, is being considered a major setback in tackling these diseases. Fortunately, there has been tremendous research done in the last few decades examining the effects of dietary patterns on chronic diseases. This information is easily available to physicians online.

Dietary Approaches to Stop Hypertension (DASH) diet originated in the 1990s. In 1992, the National Institute of Health (NIH) started funding for several research projects to see if specific dietary interventions were useful in treating hypertension. Subjects included in the study were advised to follow just the dietary interventions and not include any other lifestyle modifications to avoid any confounding factors. They found that only the dietary intervention alone was able to decrease systolic Blood Pressure by about 6 to 11 mm Hg. This effect was seen both in hypertensive as well as normotensive people. Based on these results, in some instances, DASH has been advocated as the first-line pharmacologic therapy along with lifestyle modification.

What does this diet include?

DASH promotes the consumption of vegetables and fruits, lean meat and dairy products, and the inclusion of micronutrients in the menu. It also advocates the reduction of sodium in the diet to about 1500 mg/day. DASH emphasizes on consumption of minimally processed and fresh food. DASH diet has many similarities to some of the other dietary patterns which are promoted for cardiovascular health. DASH diet is a culmination of the ancient and modern world. It has been derived by scientists based on certain ancient dietary principles and has been tailored to target some of the leading killers of modern society.

A typical serving guide for a patient following the DASH diet is as follows:

- Vegetables: about five servings per day
- Fruits: about five meals per day

- Carbohydrates: about seven servings per day

- Low-fat dairy products: about two servings per day

- Lean meat products: about two or fewer servings per day

- Nuts and seeds: 2 to 3 times per week

Following is a closer look at these recommendations.

❖ **Carbohydrates**

Carbohydrates in the diet are mainly composed of cellulose and starches. The human body cannot digest cellulose. It is mainly present in plant fiber. Healthy starches or "carbs" have to be included in the diet, not just for the energy supply but also for the protective micronutrients. Low carb diets are not as healthy as that may lead to either decreased caloric intake than recommended or consumption of unhealthy fats as a substitute.

Healthy carbohydrates included under DASH include:

- Green leafy vegetables: kale, broccoli, spinach, collards, mustards

- Whole grains: cracked wheat, millets, oats

- Low glycemic index fruits

- Legumes and beans

Fats

Fats have been a prime suspect for some time now, in the development of the chronic disease epidemic. However, research has now shown otherwise. Fats are now classified as good fats and bad fats.

Good fats prevent inflammation, provide essential fatty acids, and promote overall health. These fats, when consumed in moderation, have shown an increase in HDL and lowering of small dense LDL particles. Some of the sources of good fats also included in DASH include:

- ✓ Olive oil
- ✓ Avocados
- ✓ Nuts
- ✓ Hempseeds
- ✓ Flax seeds

Fish rich in omega-3 fatty acids

Bad fats, which include margarine, vegetable shortenings, partially hydrogenated vegetable oils, cause an increase in small LDL particles, which promote atherogenesis.

Fats are a highly condensed source of energy and therefore have to be consumed in moderation. The serving sizes are much smaller than those for other nutrients on the DASH recommendations.

Proteins

DASH recommends more servings of plant proteins like legumes, soy products, nuts, and seeds. Animal protein in the diet should mainly compose of lean meats, low-fat dairy, eggs, and fish.

Processed and cured meats are not recommended as they have shown to cause hypertension and also contain carcinogens.

DASH diet also talks about the inclusion of certain foods that are rich in potassium, calcium, and magnesium as these prevent endothelial dysfunction and promote endothelial, smooth muscle relaxation. Some of the foods rich in potassium include bananas, oranges, and spinach. Calcium is rich in dairy products and green leafy vegetables. Magnesium is present in a variety of whole grains, leafy vegetables, nuts, and seeds.

Several studies have shown that the DASH diet helps lower blood glucose levels, triglycerides, LDL-C, and insulin resistance. This makes the DASH diet a very important adjunct to pharmacological therapy in metabolic syndromes, a major epidemic in this country. It also has been a successful tool in weight management. In certain populations, adherence to the DASH diet has shown significant improvements in control of type 2 diabetes. It is a preferred diet in patients with heart failure due to its emphasis on the reduction of dietary sodium and encouraging the intake of potassium, magnesium, and calcium.

DASH diet has also shown a reduction in the incidence of colorectal cancer, mainly in the white population. DASH diet has also been proven in multiple studies to have lowered all-cause mortality in adults.

Based on these studies, it is safe to say that when combined with pharmacological intervention, DASH can be a very useful tool for physicians to tackle these diseases more efficiently. When compared to some other diet patterns, it has an added advantage of having clear guidelines on the serving sizes and food groups, which makes it easier for the physicians to prescribe and monitor their patient's improvement.

The DASH diet is a nutritionally based approach to prevent and control hypertension. The diet has been tested in several clinical trials and has been shown to lower cholesterol, saturated fats, and blood pressure. The DASH diet has been recommended as the best diet to help people who would like to lose maintain a healthy weight and lower the blood pressure. The key fact is that this diet needs to be promoted to patients. Besides physicians, both nurses and pharmacists play a key role in educating patients about the benefits of this diet. Just prior to discharge, nurses are in a prime position to educate all patients and their families about the DASH diet and its benefits. Similarly, when patients visit a pharmacy, the pharmacist should educate the patient about the DASH diet. The most important feature about the DASH diet is it requires a change in lifestyle and adopt a healthy way to eat. In addition, patients should be urged to stop smoking, abstain from alcohol, and do some physical activity on a regular basis.

DASH Diet and High Blood Pressure

One of the steps your doctor may recommend to lower your high blood pressure is to start using the DASH diet.

DASH stands for Dietary Approaches to Stop Hypertension. The diet is simple:

- Eat more fruits, vegetables, and low-fat dairy foods
- Cut back on foods that are high in saturated fat, cholesterol, and trans fats
- Eat more whole-grain foods, fish, poultry, and nuts
- Limit sodium, sweets, sugary drinks, and red meats

In research studies, people who were on the DASH diet lowered their blood pressure within 2 weeks.

Another diet -- DASH-Sodium -- calls for cutting back sodium to 1,500 milligrams a day (about 2/3 teaspoon). Studies of people on the DASH-Sodium plan lowered their blood pressure as well.

Starting the DASH Diet

The DASH diet calls for a certain number of servings daily from various food groups. The number of servings you re☐uire may vary, depending on how many calories you need per day.

You can make gradual changes. For instance, start by limiting yourself to 2,400 milligrams of sodium per day (about 1 teaspoon). Then, once your body has adjusted to the diet, cut back to 1,500 milligrams of sodium per day (about 2/3 teaspoon). These amounts include all sodium eaten, including sodium in food products as well as in what you cook with or add at the table.

Dash Diet Tips

1. Add a serving of vegetables at lunch and at dinner.
2. Add a serving of fruit to your meals or as a snack. Canned and dried fruits are easy to use, but check that they don't have added sugar.
3. Use only half your typical serving of butter, margarine, or salad dressing, and use low-fat or fat-free condiments.
4. Drink low-fat or skim dairy products any time you would normally use full-fat or cream.

5. Limit meat to 6 ounces a day. Make some meals vegetarian.

6. Add more vegetables and dry beans to your diet.

Instead of snacking on chips or sweets, eat unsalted pretzels or nuts, raisins, low-fat and fat-free yogurt, frozen yogurt, unsalted plain popcorn with no butter, and raw vegetables.

Staying on the DASH Diet

The DASH diet suggests getting:

- Grains: 7-8 daily servings
- Vegetables: 4-5 daily servings
- Fruits: 4-5 daily servings
- Low-fat or fat-free dairy products: 2-3 daily servings
- Meat, poultry, and fish: 2 or less daily servings
- Nuts, seeds, and dry beans: 4-5 servings per week
- Fats and oils: 2-3 daily servings
- Sweets: try to limit to less than 5 servings per week

How Much Is a Serving?

When you're trying to follow a healthy eating plan, it helps to know how much of a certain kind of food is considered a "serving." One serving is:

- ✓ 1/2 cup cooked rice or pasta
- ✓ 1 slice bread
- ✓ 1 cup raw vegetables or fruit
- ✓ 1/2 cup cooked veggies or fruit
- ✓ 8 ounces of milk
- ✓ 1 teaspoon of olive oil (or any other oil)
- ✓ 3 ounces cooked meat
- ✓ 3 ounces tofu

CHAPTER FIVE

HOW TO MAKE DASH DIET YOUR HABIT

Beyond reducing blood pressure, the DASH diet offers a number of potential benefits, including weight loss and reduced cancer risk. However, you shouldn't expect DASH to help you shed weight on its own — as it was designed fundamentally to lower blood pressure. Weight loss may simply be an added perk.

The diet impacts your body in several ways.

1) Lowers Blood Pressure

Blood pressure is a measure of the force put on your blood vessels and organs as your blood passes through them. It's counted in two numbers:

- Systolic pressure: The pressure in your blood vessels when your heart beats.
- Diastolic pressure: The pressure in your blood vessels between heartbeats, when your heart is at rest.

Normal blood pressure for adults is a systolic pressure below 120 mmHg and a diastolic pressure below 80 mmHg. This is normally written with the systolic blood pressure above the diastolic pressure, like this: 120/80.

People with a blood pressure reading of 140/90 are considered to have high blood pressure. Interestingly, the DASH diet demonstrably lowers blood pressure in both healthy people and those with high blood pressure.

In studies, people on the DASH diet still experienced lower blood pressure even if they didn't lose weight or restrict salt intake.

However, when sodium intake was restricted, the DASH diet lowered blood pressure even further. In fact, the greatest reductions in blood pressure were seen in people with the lowest salt consumption.

These low-salt DASH diet results were most impressive in people who already had high blood pressure, reducing systolic blood pressure by an average of 12 mmHg and diastolic blood pressure by 5 mmHg. In people with normal blood pressure, it reduced systolic blood pressure by 4 mmHg and diastolic by 2 mmHg.

This is in line with other studies which reveal that restricting salt intake can reduce blood pressure — especially in those who have high blood pressure. Keep in mind that a decrease in blood pressure does not always translate to a decreased risk of heart disease.

2) May Aid Weight Loss

You will likely experience lower blood pressure on the DASH diet whether or not you lose weight. However, if you already have high blood pressure, chances are you have been advised to lose weight.

This is because the more you weigh, the higher your blood pressure is likely to be. Additionally, losing weight has been shown to lower blood pressure. Some studies suggest that people can lose weight on the DASH diet.

However, those who have lost weight on the DASH diet have been in a controlled calorie deficit — meaning they were told to eat fewer calories than they were expending.

Given that the DASH diet cuts out a lot of high-fat, sugary foods, people may find that they automatically reduce their calorie intake and lose weight. Other people may have to consciously restrict their intake. Either way, if you want to lose weight on the DASH diet, you'll still need to go on a calorie-reduced diet.

Other Potential Health Benefits

DASH may also affect other areas of health. The diet:

Decreases cancer risk: A recent review indicated that people following the DASH diet had a lower risk of some cancers, including colorectal and breast cancer. Lowers metabolic syndrome risk: Some studies note that the DASH diet reduces your risk of metabolic syndrome by up to 81%.

Lowers diabetes risk: The diet has been linked to a lower risk of type 2 diabetes. Some studies demonstrate that it can improve insulin resistance as well.

Decreases heart disease risk: In one recent review in women, following a DASH-like diet was associated with a 20% lower risk of heart disease and a 29% lower risk of stroke.

Many of these protective effects are attributed to the diet's high fruit and vegetable content. In general, eating more fruits and vegetables can help reduce risk of disease.

<u>Restricting Salt Too Much Is Not Good for You</u>

Eating too little salt has been linked to health problems, such as an increased risk of heart disease, insulin resistance and fluid retention.

The low-salt version of the DASH diet recommends that people eat no more than 3/4 teaspoon (1,500 mg) of sodium per day. However, it's unclear whether there are any benefits to reducing salt intake this low — even in people with high blood pressure.

In fact, a recent review found no link between salt intake and risk of death from heart disease, despite the fact that lowering salt intake caused a modest reduction in blood pressure. However, because most people eat too much salt, lowering your salt intake from very high amounts of 2–2.5 teaspoons (10–12 grams) a day to 1–1.25 teaspoons (5–6 grams) a day may be beneficial.

This target can be achieved easily by reducing the amount of highly processed food in your diet and eating mostly whole foods.

How to Make Your Diet More DASH-Like

Because there are no set foods on the DASH diet, you can adapt your current diet to the DASH guidelines by doing the following:

- Eat more vegetables and fruits.
- Swap refined grains for whole grains.
- Choose fat-free or low-fat dairy products.
- Choose lean protein sources like fish, poultry and beans.
- Cook with vegetable oils.
- Limit your intake of foods high in added sugars, like soda and candy.
- Limit your intake of foods high in saturated fats like fatty meats, full-fat dairy and oils like coconut and palm oil.

Outside of measured fresh fruit juice portions, this diet recommends you stick to low-calorie drinks like water, tea and coffee.

Frequently Asked Questions

If you're thinking about trying DASH to lower your blood pressure, you might have a few questions about other aspects of your lifestyle.

The most commonly asked □uestions are addressed below.

Can I Drink Coffee on the DASH Diet?

The DASH diet doesn't prescribe specific guidelines for coffee. However, some people worry that caffeinated beverages like coffee may increase their blood pressure. It's well known that caffeine can cause a short-term increase in blood pressure.

Furthermore, this rise is greater in people with high blood pressure. However, a recent review claimed that this popular beverage doesn't increase the long-term risk of high blood pressure or heart disease — even though it caused a short-term (1–3 hours) increase in blood pressure.

For most healthy people with normal blood pressure, 3–4 regular cups of coffee per day are considered safe. Keep in mind that the slight rise in blood pressure (5–10 mm Hg) caused by caffeine means that people who already have high blood pressure probably need to be more careful with their coffee consumption.

Do I Need to Exercise on the DASH Diet?

The DASH diet is even more effective at lowering blood pressure when paired with physical activity. Given the independent benefits of exercise on health, this is not surprising. It's recommended to do 30 minutes of moderate activity most days, and it's important to choose something you enjoy — this way, you will be more likely to keep it up.

Examples of moderate activity include:

- ✓ Brisk walking (15 minutes per mile or 9 minutes per kilometer)
- ✓ Running (10 minutes per mile or 6 minutes per kilometer)
- ✓ Cycling (6 minutes per mile or 4 minutes per kilometer)

✓ Swimming laps (20 minutes)

✓ Housework (60 minutes)

Can I Drink Alcohol on the DASH Diet?

Drinking too much alcohol can increase your blood pressure. In fact, regularly drinking more than 3 drinks per day has been linked to an increased risk of high blood pressure and heart disease.

On the DASH diet, you should drink alcohol sparingly and not exceed official guidelines — 2 or fewer drinks per day for men and 1 or fewer for women. The DASH diet may be an easy and effective way to reduce blood pressure.

However, keep in mind that cutting daily salt intake to 3/4 teaspoon (1,500 mg) or less has not been linked to any hard health benefits — such as a reduced risk of heart disease — despite the fact that it can lower blood pressure. Moreover, the DASH diet is very similar to the standard low-fat diet, which large controlled trials have not shown to reduce the risk of death by heart disease.

Healthy individuals may have little reason to follow this diet. Nevertheless, if you have high blood pressure or think you may be sensitive to salt, DASH may be a good choice for you.

CHAPTER SIX

SIMPLE EXERCISES TO FOLLOW WITH THE

DIET

In older adults with cognitive impairment and cardiovascular risk factors, aerobic exercise improved executive function, a set of complex mental processes that are important for attention, organization, planning, decision-making, and regulating emotions. Researchers also found that the greatest improvement in executive function was seen in participants who combined aerobic exercise with the Dietary Approaches to Stop Hypertension (DASH) diet.

These findings come from the Exercise and Nutritional Interventions for Neurocognitive Health Enhancement (ENLIGHTEN) study, a randomized controlled trial that included 160 sedentary men and women over the age of 55 who had cognitive impairments without dementia, and risk factors for cardiovascular disease. Participants were randomly assigned to one of four groups: aerobic exercise alone, DASH diet alone, aerobic exercise combined with DASH diet, or a control group that just received health education. The intervention lasted six months.

At baseline, participants had executive function comparable to that of people in their early 90s, approximately 28 years older than their chronological age. Participants who engaged in aerobic exercise showed significant improvement in executive function, while those in the DASH diet alone did not. Interestingly, however, the greatest improvement in executive function was seen in participants who engaged in both aerobic exercise and the DASH diet. After six months, the exercise plus DASH diet group showed improvement in executive function that was equivalent to taking off 8.8 years. In contrast, the health education control group had performance that was worse than their baseline. Although positive effects were seen in executive function, none of the study interventions resulted in significant improvement in memory or language fluency.

Participants in the aerobic exercise group exercised three times a week for six months. The first 10 minutes consisted of warm-up exercises and these were followed by 30 minutes of continuous walking or stationary cycling.

The DASH diet group received instructions on modifying their diet. A series of half-hour sessions were conducted by a nutritionist weekly for the first three months, then biweekly for the subsequent three months. The DASH diet plan emphasizes high intakes of fruits, vegetables, whole grains, and low-fat dairy products, as well as increased potassium and reduced sodium intake. Participants in the DASH diet group were asked not to exercise.

Participants in the exercise plus DASH diet received both interventions as described above. Those in the health education (control) group received half-hour calls from a health educator who discussed cardiovascular health-related topics, weekly for the first three months, then biweekly for the subsequent three months.

Although the precise mechanisms underlying the benefits of exercise on executive function are not clear, increased aerobic fitness, reduced cardiovascular disease risk, and reduced sodium intake were all associated with improved executive function. There is growing evidence that multi-component lifestyle changes (e.g., exercise, nutrition, cognitive training, and management of risk factors) may protect people from cognitive decline. Problems with blood vessels, including high blood pressure, diabetes, and high cholesterol have all been associated with cognitive decline and dementia, while exercise and a healthy diet counter these conditions. In addition, both exercise and a healthy diet increase a protein called BDNF that supports the growth and survival of brain cells. Findings from this randomized clinical trial are consistent with the seven steps we recommend for brain health.

When you think of exercise, you may imagine strenuous activities such as running or biking — the ones that make you breathe hard, turn flush and drip with sweat. But aerobic activity is only one type of exercise, and although it is critical for boosting fitness, there are actually three other types of exercise that are also important: strength training, balance training and flexibility training.

"While aerobic exercise is very important, it's not as effective for overall health" when done alone compared with when people include all four types of exercise in their routine.

> ➢ **Aerobic exercise**

Aerobic exercises, such as running, swimming or dancing, are activities that work your cardiovascular system — they get your heart rate up and make you breathe harder. This type of exercise can reduce the risk of cardiovascular disease, type 2 diabetes and high blood pressure, and may even lower the risk of cancer.

> ➢ **Strength exercise**

Strength exercises, such as weight lifting, push-ups and crunches, work your muscles by using resistance (like a dumbbell or your own body weight.) This type of exercise increases lean muscle mass, which is particularly important for weight loss, because lean muscle burns more calories than other types of tissue. Full story: Here's what you need to know about strength training.

> ➢ **Balance exercise**

Balance exercises improve your ability to control and stabilize your body's position. This type of exercise is particularly important for older adults, because balance gets worse with age.But balance exercises can be beneficial for everyone, including people who have gained or lost a lot of weight or those who become pregnant, which can throw off your center of gravity.

> ➢ **Flexibility exercise**

Flexibility exercises stretch your muscles and may improve your range of motion at your joints. They can improve your flexibility, and reduce your risk of injury during sports and other activities.

Ideally, you should include all four types of exercise in your workouts. But that doesn't mean you have to do four separate workouts, Drew said. You can combine some exercises together, like strength and balance training. For example, you could do bicep curls while standing on one leg. Some workouts, such as yoga, incorporate strength, flexibility and balance exercises.

Set Yourself Up for Success with the DASH Diet

Creating and practicing a new routine, such as the Dietary Approaches to Stop Hypertension (DASH) diet, is part of establishing a new habit. If your diet is low in fruits and vegetables and high in salt and fat right now, you can't expect to do a complete turnaround overnight. You have to establish a few small goals at a time and work on those goals until they become new habits.

After you adopt a few new habits, you can move on to the next few goals. You can successfully follow a DASH diet plan if you Make a commitment to change your habits for the long haul, not just your food and beverage intake.

Are open to learning more about how your body works and why diet truly has an impact on health. Replace overeating behaviors with other strategies for coping with stress, boredom, and other situations where emotions rule eating.

- Stay open-minded about trying new foods.
- Understand that modifying your diet to include DASH diet principles isn't a quick fix, nor are the overall lifestyle changes you'll make.
- Realize that you'll have setbacks — and that you can forgive yourself and move on.
- Seek a support system to help you meet your eating and exercise goals.

Of course, before you make any changes in your diet or lifestyle, you have to be in the "action phase" of readiness, which is the fourth stage of the classic five-stage model for successful behavioral change:

❖ **Precontemplation:**

In this stage, you're not even thinking about changing your diet or lifestyle, and you may not even realize that you have a problem (for instance, if you're overweight or your doctor has told you that your diet is affecting your health).

❖ **Contemplation:**

During this stage, you're willing to consider making some changes, but you ay be on the fence.

❖ **Determination:**

The fact that you're holding this book in your hands probably means you're at least in the determination stage. You've thought about it, you're making a plan, and you're ready to commit to some action.

❖ **Action:**

In this stage, you may also be sharing your goals with others, making you more accountable. During this stage, you continue to work on your plan by setting goals and tracking progress. Success breeds success!

The success you have (whether it's lower blood pressure, weight loss, lower blood cholesterol, or just feeling better) is a huge motivator to keep on track. You may be in the action stage for at least three to six months, and this leads to maintenance.

❖ **Maintenance:**

This stage is a lifelong endeavor where you address the ups and downs and get through situations that are challenging (vacations, holidays, and other special occasions).

Generally, most people go through each stage and often have setbacks along the way. Provided you recover from them, those setbacks are A-OK because the DASH diet isn't a ꓺuick-fix fad diet; it's a diet to adopt for a lifetime of healthy eating.

Your long-term goal is to develop a healthy eating and exercise plan that you can live with for the rest of your life. You can do this by making gradual changes, following the dietary guidelines at least 80 percent of the time, and recovering quickly when you do get off track.

Setting up an appointment with a registered dietitian/nutritionist (RDN) can help you get started with a plan that's just right for you. An RDN will review your personal medical history and provide a nutrition assessment and personalized plan. Give your local medical center or your primary physician a call about referral to a local RDN.

CHAPTER SEVEN

14 DAYS DASH DIET MEAL PLAN

If you feel like your healthy habits have gotten off track, this simple take on a clean-eating meal plan can help you get back to the eating habits that help you feel your best. Over the course of this 14-day diet plan, you'll get your fill of healthy whole foods-some that you'll prep from scratch and others that you can buy from the store.

The meals and snacks in this plan will have you feeling energized, satisfied and good about what's on your plate. And at 1,200 calories, this diet meal plan will set you up to lose upwards of 4 pounds over the 2 weeks.

Clean-Eating Meal Plan for Beginners

If you're new to clean eating, the premise is simple—and following a meal plan (or simply using it for inspiration) can make it even easier to understand what it's all about. Clean-eating is a great way to up your intake of good-for-you foods (like whole grains, lean protein, healthy fats and plenty of fruits and veggies), while limiting the stuff that can make you feel not-so-great in large amounts (think refined carbs, alcohol, added sugars and hydrogenated fats).

While all foods can be part of a healthy diet, sometimes you just need to hit reset and focus on eating more of the healthy foods you may be skimping on. With 14 days of wholesome meals and snacks, this easy-to-follow clean-eating meal plan is a great way get more of those good for you foods.

If 14 days feel like too much, start with our 3-Day Clean Eating Kick-Start Meal Plan and go from there. Once you conquer this 14-day plan, try our Clean-Eating Challenge for 30 days, where you can plan to eat tons of delicious clean-eating foods, like what you'll find in this meal plan.

Week 1

How to Meal Prep Your Week of Meals:

A little prep at the beginning of the week goes a long way to make your week ahead easy.

Make a double batch of the Lemon-Tahini Dressing. You'll use it throughout the week for lunch and dinner. Store in this classic glass salad dressing container. (To buy: amazon.com, $8.29)

Cook a double batch of the Easy Brown Rice to use throughout the week. Store in a large glass meal-prep container. (To buy: amazon.com, $38) Because Day 1's dinner—the Kale Salad with Beets & Wild Rice—calls for wild rice, you can choose to either prep a bigger batch of wild rice or swap in brown rice in the recipe so you're not having to make two different rices.

❖ **Day 1**

Breakfast (287 calories)

- 1 serving Muesli with Raspberries

Clean-Eating Shopping Tip: When buying muesli, look for a brand that doesn't have added sugars, which take away from the healthy goodness of this whole-grain breakfast.

A.M. Snack (62 calories)

- 1 medium orange

Lunch (360 calories)

- 4 cups White Bean & Veggie Salad

P.M. Snack (95 calories)

- 1 medium apple

Dinner (420 calories)

- 4 cups (1 1/2 servings) Kale Salad with Beets & Wild Rice
- 1 serving Balsamic-Dijon Chicken

Meal-Prep Tip: Save 1 serving Balsamic-Dijon Chicken (1/2 breast) for lunch of Day 2.

Daily Totals: 1,224 calories, 61 g protein, 153 g carbohydrates, 40 g fiber, 47 g fat, 1,400 mg sodium.

❖ **Day 2**

Breakfast (270 calories)

- 1 serving Avocado-Egg Toast

Clean-Eating Shopping Tip: Use sprouted-grain bread as your bread for these next two weeks as it's made without added sugars, unlike many store-bought breads. Also, if you plan to top your egg toast with hot sauce, look for a brand that's made without added sugars.

A.M. Snack (101 calories)

- 1 medium pear

Lunch (353 calories)

- 2 cups mixed greens
- 1/2 cup chopped cucumber
- 1/2 Balsamic-Dijon Chicken breast, chopped
- 2 Tbsp. Lemon-Tahini Dressing
- Tbsp. sunflower seeds

Combine greens, cucumber and chicken and top with dressing and sunflower seeds.

If you're taking this salad to go, pack it up in this handy meal-prep container, specifically made to keep your greens fresh and dressing separate until you're ready to eat. Buy It! amazon.com, $35 for a two-pack.

P.M. Snack (62 calories)

- 1 medium orange

Dinner (439 calories)

- 1 serving cup S␣uash & Red Lentil Curry
- 1/2 cup Easy Brown Rice

Meal-Prep Tip: Save a 1 cup serving of rice to have for dinner on Day 3.

Daily Totals: 1,225 calories, 63 g protein, 147 g carbohydrates, 33 g fiber, 46 g fat, 1,965 mg sodium.

❖ **Day 3**

Breakfast (287 calories)

- 1 serving Muesli with Raspberries

A.M. Snack (62 calories)

- 1 medium orange

Lunch (326 calories)

- 1 serving cups Squash & Red Lentil Curry

P.M. Snack (92 calories)

- 12 almonds

Dinner (439 calories)

- 1 serving Asian Tilapia with Stir-Fried Green Beans
- 1 cup Easy Brown Rice

Daily Totals: 1,206 calories, 62 g protein, 174 g carbohydrates, 37 g fiber, 48 g fat, 1,444 mg sodium.

❖ **Day 4**

Breakfast (257 calories)

- 1/2 cup rolled oats, cooked in 1 cup milk
- 1 medium plum, chopped

Cook oats and top with plum and a pinch of cinnamon.

A.M. Snack (95 calories)

- 1 medium apple

Lunch (325 calories)

- 1 serving Veggie & Hummus Sandwich

Clean-Eating Shopping Tip: Double-check the ingredient list on hummus to make sure you're choosing one without added sugars or excess sodium. You can also try making your own. EatingWell's Garlic Hummus is both easy and delicious.

P.M. Snack (105 calories)

- 1 medium banana

Dinner (432 calories)

- 1 serving Sheet-Pan Chicken & Brussels Sprouts

- 1 1/2 cups mixed greens dressed with 2 Tbsp. Lemon-Tahini Dressing

Daily Totals: 1,214 calories, 58 g protein, 166 g carbohydrates, 32 g fiber, 41 g fat, 1,553 mg sodium.

❖ **Day 5**

Breakfast (290 calories)

- 1 serving Peanut Butter-Banana Cinnamon Toast

Clean-Eating Shopping Tip: When choosing a store-bought peanut butter, avoid brands with added sugars and trans fats. Read more about choosing a healthy peanut butter.

A.M. Snack (32 calories)

- 1/2 cup raspberries

Lunch (360 calories)

- 4 cups White Bean & Veggie Salad

Dinner (543 calories)

- 1 serving Pork Chops with Garlicky Broccoli

Daily Totals: 1,225 calories, 54 g protein, 102 g carbohydrates, 30 g fiber, 71 g fat, 1,175 mg sodium.

❖ **Day 6**

Breakfast (257 calories)

- 1/2 cup rolled oats, cooked in 1 cup milk
- 1 medium plum, chopped

Cook oats and top with plum and a pinch of cinnamon.

A.M. Snack (101 calories)

- 1 medium pear

Lunch (325 calories)

- 1 serving Veggie & Hummus Sandwich

P.M. Snack (62 calories)

- 1 medium orange

Dinner (543 calories)

- 1 serving Cauliflower Rice-Stuffed Peppers
- 2 cups mixed greens dressed with 1 Tbsp. Citrus Vinaigrette

Meal-Prep Tip: You'll use the remaining Citrus Vinaigrette next week.

Daily Totals: 1,203 calories, 57g protein, 146 g carbohydrates, 31 g fiber, 49 g fat, 1,120 mg sodium.

❖ **Day 7**

Breakfast (307 calories)

- 2 cups Jason Mraz's Avocado Green Smoothie

A.M. Snack (35 calories)

- 1 clementine

Lunch (352 calories)

- 2 1/4 cup Tomato, Cucumber & White-Bean Salad with Basil Vinaigrette
- 1 slice sprouted-grain bread, toasted and topped with 1 Tbsp. hummus

Meal-Prep Tip: Save a serving of the Tomato, Cucumber & White-Bean Salad with Basil Vinaigrette to have for lunch on Day 10. Store the dressing separately.

P.M. Snack (30 calories)

- 1 plum

Dinner (490 calories)

- 1 1/2 cups Mexican Cabbage Soup
- 2 cups No-Cook Black Bean Salad

Meal-Prep Tip: Save a 1-cup serving of the No-Cook Black Bean Salad to have for lunch on Day 9. Store the dressing separately and wait to add until ready to eat. Pack up 2 servings of the Mexican Cabbage Soup in a leak-proof container (To buy: amazon.com, $7.19 for 1) to have for lunch on Days 9 & 12.

Daily Totals: 1,214 calories, 35 g protein, 163 g carbohydrates, 48 g fiber, 55 g fat, 1,365 mg sodium.

Week 2

How to Meal Prep Your Week of Meals:

A little prep at the beginning of the week goes a long way to make your week ahead easy.

Make a batch of the Meal-Prep Sheet-Pan Chicken Thighs and Basic Quinoa when preparing the Greek Kale Salad with Quinoa & Chicken recipe for dinner on Day 8. This way, you'll have leftover chicken and □uinoa to use during the week. Store leftovers of the chicken and □uinoa separately in large glass meal-prep containers. (To buy: amazon.com, $38)

❖ **Day 8**

Breakfast (338 calories)

- 1 serving Scrambled Eggs with Vegetables

A.M. Snack (119 calories)

- 1/4 cup hummus
- 1 cup sliced cucumber

Lunch (325 calories)

- 1 serving Veggie & Hummus Sandwich

P.M. Snack (30 calories)

- 1 plum

Dinner (302 calories)

- 1 serving Greek Kale Salad with Quinoa & Chicken

Evening Snack (102 calories)

- 1 serving Broiled Mango

Daily Totals: 1,216 calories, 58 g protein, 121 g carbohydrates, 26 g fiber, 60 g fat, 1,816 mg sodium.

❖ **Day 9**

Breakfast (307 calories)

- 2 cups Jason Mraz's Avocado Green Smoothie

A.M. Snack (35 calories)

- 1 clementine

Lunch (328 calories)

- 1 1/2 cups Mexican Cabbage Soup
- 1 cup No-Cook Black Bean Salad

P.M. Snack (92 calories)

- 3/4 cup Kiwi & Mango with Fresh Lime Zest

Dinner (453 calories)

- 1 cup riced cauliflower, heated
- 1 serving Soy-Lime Roasted Tofu
- 2 cups Colorful Roasted Sheet-Pan Veggies
- 1 Tbsp. Citrus Vinaigrette

Top riced cauliflower with tofu, veggies and drizzle with the vinaigrette.

Daily Totals: 1,216 calories, 44 g protein, 149 g carbohydrates, 42 g fiber, 59 g fat, 1,248 mg sodium.

- ❖ **Day 10**

Breakfast (290 calories)

- 1 serving Peanut Butter-Banana Cinnamon Toast

A.M. Snack (64 calories)

- 1 cup raspberries

Lunch (370 calories)

- 1 serving Chicken & Apple Kale Wraps

P.M. Snack (92 calories)

- 1 plum
- 8 almonds

Dinner (402 calories)

- 1 serving Panko-Crusted Pork Chops with Asian Slaw

Daily Totals: 1,217 calories, 72 g protein, 127 g carbohydrates, 29 g fiber, 50 g fat, 1,133 mg sodium.

❖ **Day 11**

Breakfast (270 calories)

- 1 serving Avocado-Egg Toast

A.M. Snack (64 calories)

- 1 cup raspberries

Lunch (302 calories)

- 1 serving Greek Kale Salad with Quinoa & Chicken

P.M. Snack (95 calories)

- 1 medium apple

Dinner (478 calories)

- 1 serving Salmon & Asparagus with Lemon-Garlic Butter Sauce
- 1 cup Basic Quinoa

Meal-Prep Tip: Cook a hard-boiled egg tonight so it's ready for your P.M. Snack on Day 12.

Daily Totals: 1,209 calories, 68 g protein, 128 g carbohydrates, 28 g fiber, 50 g fat, 1,233 mg sodium.

❖ **Day 12**

Breakfast (290 calories)

- 1 serving Peanut Butter-Banana Cinnamon Toast

A.M. Snack (96 calories)

- 1 clementine
- 8 almonds

Lunch (344 calories)

- 1 1/2 cups Mexican Cabbage Soup
- 2 cups mixed greens
- 1 Tbsp. Citrus Vinaigrette
- 2 Tbsp. sunflower seeds

Toss greens in vinaigrette. Top with sunflower seeds.

P.M. Snack (78 calories)

- 1 hard-boiled egg, seasoned with a pinch each of salt and pepper

Dinner (408 calories)

- 1 serving Spaghetti Squash & Meatballs

Daily Totals: 1,216 calories, 60 g protein, 124 g carbohydrates, 30 g fiber, 56 g fat, 1,463 mg sodium.

❖ **Day 13**

Breakfast (264 calories)

- 1 cup nonfat plain Greek yogurt
- 1/4 cup muesli
- 1/4 cup blueberries

A.M. Snack (70 calories)

- 2 clementines

Lunch (325 calories)

- 1 serving Veggie & Hummus Sandwich

P.M. Snack (95 calories)

- 1 medium apple

Dinner (446 calories)

- 1 serving Zucchini Noodles with Avocado Pesto & Shrimp

Daily Totals: 1,200 calories, 68 g protein, 133 g carbohydrates, 31 g fiber, 52 g fat, 1,102 mg sodium.

❖ **Day 14**

Breakfast (270 calories)

- 1 serving Avocado-Egg Toast

A.M. Snack (70 calories)

- 2 clementines

Lunch (378 calories)

- 2 1/4 cup Tomato, Cucumber & White-Bean Salad with Basil Vinaigrette
- 1 slice sprouted-grain bread, toasted and topped with 2 Tbsp. hummus

P.M. Snack (30 calories)

- 1 plum

Dinner (458 calories)

- 1 serving Fish with Coconut-Shallot Sauce
- 1/2 cup Basic Quinoa
- 2 cups mixed greens topped with 1 Tbsp. Citrus Vinaigrette

Daily Totals: 1,207 calories, 61 g protein, 113 g carbohydrates, 27 g fiber, 60 g fat, 1,146 mg sodium.

CHAPTER EIGHT

DASH BREAKFAST RECIPES

The purpose-created Dietary Approaches to Stop Hypertension (DASH) diet is designed to help you lower your blood pressure naturally, as part of an overall plan to reduce your risk of deadly heart disease. Heart disease is the number one killer of men and women in the developed world, and unlike the second leading cause—cancer—there are concrete steps one can take to dramatically reduce the risk of falling victim to this killer.

That's because many of the risk factors for heart disease are actually under our control. They include engaging in adequate exercise on a routine basis, avoiding obesity, and eating a healthful diet. Simply cutting added sugars from the diet, for example, can slash your risk. Adding more fruits, vegetables, and whole grains—and eating less processed and red meat—can also affect your risk profile significantly. Too much sugar and too much consumption of meat have been linked to poorer health.

Conversely, replacing these foods with more healthful alternatives can be beneficial.

Bigger is Better

Recent research suggests that for people seeking to lose (or control) body weight, eating a big breakfast, a more modest lunch, and having the lightest meal of the day at dinner time is an eating pattern associated with better weight loss and control. It seems we fare best when we consume the bulk of our daily calories early in the day.

This flies in the face of most Americans' experiences and practices. We tend to eat breakfast on the run, if at all, and save the big meal for the end of the day. There is a better way. Why not try eating the majority of your calories in the morning, and give yourself time to enjoy your feast?

Here's an important tip: Never, ever, skip breakfast. It's counter-productive, because it sets you up for overeating later in the day. Here are some other important tips that can add up to better health success.

Banish Sugar- and Artificially-Sweetened Beverages

Wave bye bye to soft drinks. Even zero-calorie ones. Or perhaps, especially no-calorie, diet soft drinks. In recent years, consumption of these "diet" drinks has been linked to greater weight gain, not less. And more recently, researchers have noted a link between intake of these beverages and a greater risk of both stroke and dementia. That includes Alzheimer's disease. Yes, you read that right: artificially-sweetened drink consumption is associated with a significantly greater risk of developing Alzheimer's disease. Even sugar-laced soft drinks aren't that dangerous.

DASH Breakfast

To design the DASH breakfast that works best for you, keep several points in mind. There is an emphasis on reducing sodium intake. That means you should limit table salt during cooking, and use restraint at the table. However, not everyone is "salt sensitive," and thus not everyone will experience blood pressure reductions due to limitations on salt in the diet. Boosting fiber, and cutting added sugars, however, should help keep blood pressure in check no matter who you are.

Another reason health experts are such a fan of the DASH diet is that it isn't restrictive and is actually pretty easy to stick with. Need proof? Check out the recipes rounded up here, for every meal of the day. Not only are they all DASH diet-compliant, they'll have your mouth watering.

1. Pineapple Protein Smoothie

Packed with protein, this breakfast smoothie recipe is guaranteed to keep you full and satisfied. Plus, pineapple is a refreshing summer treat that will help keep your bloat away.

Ingredients

- ✓ 3/4 cup milk
- ✓ 3/4 cup pineapple chunks
- ✓ 1/2 cup ice
- ✓ 3/4 cup canned chick peas (rinsed and drained)
- ✓ 2 tbsp almond butter
- ✓ 2 pitted dates
- ✓ 2 tsp ground turmeric

Directions

1. Blend all ingredients until smooth.

2. Spinach Sunshine Smoothie Bowl

Switch up your morning smoothie routine and try a smoothie bowl recipe. This satisfying dish contains lots of vitamins and minerals from the spinach, banana, and orange juice; and heart-healthy monounsaturated fats from the avocado. Plus, for added health value, you can top the bowl with blueberries, diced pineapple, ground flaxseeds, and whatever toppings you desire. What better way to cool down and treat yourself than with this blended beauty?

Ingredients

- 1 packed cup baby spinach
- 1 banana
- 1 cup orange juice
- 1/2 avocado
- 1/2 cup ice cubes
- blueberries (optional)
- diced pineapple (optional)
- ground flaxseeds (optional)

Directions

1. Process the spinach, banana, orange juice, avocado, and ice in a blender until very smooth.

2. Serve topped with blueberries, diced pineapple, and ground flaxseeds.

3. Almond Butter Berry Smoothie

Enjoy your morning fruit with a dose of nutty-flavored nutrients by blending up this delicious smoothie.

Ingredients

- ✓ 1/4 cup 1% low-fat milk
- ✓ 1/2 medium ripe banana
- ✓ 1 tbsp creamy almond butter
- ✓ 1 cup fresh or frozen raspberries
- ✓ 1/2 cup crushed ice

Directions

1. **Blend all ingredients until smooth and enjoy!**
4. **Pomegranate and Peaches Avocado Toast**

This avocado toast tastes like dessert, but with all the added health benefits. The peaches and honey add a welcomed sweetness, the ricotta feels super indulgent, and the pomegranate seeds lend a juicy, crunchy texture.

Ingredients

- ✓ 1 slice whole grain bread
- ✓ 1/2 avocado
- ✓ 1 tsp ricotta
- ✓ pomegranate seeds, small handful
- ✓ honey, drizzle

Directions

1. Toast the whole grain bread in the oven or toaster.
2. Spread avocado onto the toast, as smooth or coarse as you prefer.
3. Spread a dollop of ricotta across the avocado.
4. Drizzle a bit of honey over the avocado mixture.
5. Sprinkle pomegrante seeds on top and enjoy.
5. **Breakfast in a Jar**

Enjoy a healthy breakfast on the go with this overnight oats recipe. Simply put the ingredients in a jar in the fridge overnight and grab a spoon the next morning. This recipe can also double as a perfect afternoon pick-me-up.

Ingredients

- ✓ 1/4 cup oatmeal
- ✓ 3/4 cup kefir
- ✓ 1 tbsp chia seeds
- ✓ 2 tbsp raisins
- ✓ 1 tbsp unsweetened coconut flakes

Directions

1. Layer ingredients in a 16-ounce mason jar, close the lid, and refrigerate overnight.
2. When ready to eat, remove the jar from the fridge and give it a quick stir.

6. Avocado Egg Cups

Loaded with healthy fats, protein, and fiber, this snack is a sight to behold. Mix up the toppings to create an avocado egg cup all your own.

Ingredients

- ✓ 2 avocados, ripe
- ✓ 1/4 tsp coarse salt
- ✓ 1/4 tsp pepper
- ✓ 1/2 tsp olive oil

- ✓ 4 medium eggs
- ✓ 1 tbsp grated cheese, such as Parmesan, cheddar, or Swiss
- ✓ assorted toppings: herbs, scallions, salsa, diced tomato, crumbled bacon, Sriracha, paprika, crumbled feta

Directions

1. Heat oven to 375°F. Halve avocados lengthwise and pit. Cut a very thin slice from bottom of each avocado half so that it sits level. Where the pit was, scoop out just enough of the flesh (about ½ tbsp) to make room for an egg.
2. Place avocados on a foil-lined rimmed baking sheet. Season each with salt and pepper, and rub with olive oil.
3. Crack an egg into each cavity (some of the egg white will run over the side, but don't worry about it). Sprinkle with cheese, if using. Cover loosely with foil.
4. Bake 20 to 25 minutes, or until eggs are set to your liking. Sprinkle with toppings.

7. Daphne Sugar Break Apple and Peanut Butter Oatmeal

A dash of cinnamon adds the perfect amount of sweetness, ideal for those times when you want a break from sugar.

Ingredients

- ✓ 1 cup steel-cut oats
- ✓ 3 medium-large Granny Smith apples, cored and sliced into 1-2" chunks
- ✓ swirl of peanut butter
- ✓ pinch ground cinnamon
- ✓ 1 tbsp butter (optional)
- ✓ 4 cups water
- ✓ pinch salt

Directions

1. Cook the oats until they reach desired texture and creaminess.
2. Chop apples, toss them into the oats, and stir.
3. Add peanut butter and mix until melted and spread throughout.
4. Top with a dash of cinnamon and butter (optional) and enjoy!

8. **Sweet Potato Toast**

Sweet potato toast is rapidly becoming the next big health food to try. This bread-free alternative to toast makes your morning carbs healthier and is perfect for gluten-free eaters, too. Simply swap out your morning slice of toast for a couple of slices of sweet potato topped with your favorite flavor combinations like nut butter, hummus, or avocado. Plus, sweet potatoes are packed with antioxidants and other nutrients that keep your body healthy and slow signs of aging.

Ingredients

- ✓ sweet potato

Directions

1. Cut the sweet potato into 1/4-inch slices and pop into the toaster.
2. Top with anything you choose. Popular combinations include: nut butter with fruit, avocado, hummus, eggs, cheese, and tuna salad.

Note: Calorie count is based off of one sweet potato and does not factor in toppings. Different toppings can add anywhere from 25-383 additional calories.

9. Ulli's Granulli

This great mixture is loaded with healthy nuts, seeds, and dried fruit to spice up your breakfast. Put this mix on top of your morning Greek yogurt to enjoy a breakfast filled with protein and healthy fats.

Ingredients

- ✓ 4 cups rolled oats
- ✓ 2 cups raw cashews
- ✓ 2 cups raw walnuts
- ✓ 2 cups raw almonds
- ✓ 2 cups raw sunflower seeds
- ✓ 2 cups raw pumpkin seeds
- ✓ 3 cups unsweetened coconut flakes
- ✓ 1/2 cup maple syrup
- ✓ 1/4 cup unrefined coconut oil, plus 2 tsp for oiling the baking sheet
- ✓ pinch of sea salt
- ✓ 1/3 cup pure orange oil
- ✓ 2 cups organic raisins
- ✓ 2 cups dried cherries or cranberries

Directions

1. Preheat the oven to 300°F.

2. In a very large bowl combine the oats, nuts, seeds and coconut flakes and mix well.

3. In a smaller bowl whisk together the maple syrup, coconut oil, salt and orange oil until well combined then pour over the oat-nut mixture and mix well.

4. Spread granola on a large oiled baking sheet (do it in batches if needed) and bake for 35-40 minutes until golden brown (rotate the baking sheet halfway through for even baking).

5. Remove from oven and let cool completely before mixing with raisins and dried cherries or cranberries.

6. Store in airtight containers in the fridge to maintain extra crispiness.

10. Whole Grain Cottage Cheese Pancakes

Don't feel bad about eating pancakes for breakfast with this delicious and nutritious recipe. The addition of cottage cheese adds protein to your otherwise carb-filled pancakes which can help you keep your weight under control and keep daily cravings at bay.

Ingredients

- ✓ 1 cup oat flour
- ✓ 1/2 cup sorghum flour
- ✓ 2 tbsp teff flour
- ✓ 1/3 cup plus 1 tbsp, tapioca starch
- ✓ 1 tbsp baking powder
- ✓ 1/2 tsp salt
- ✓ 3 1/2 tsp sugar
- ✓ 1/2 tsp flax meal
- ✓ 3/4 cup buttermilk
- ✓ 1/3 cup cottage cheese
- ✓ 3 eggs
- ✓ 1/2 tsp vanilla extract
- ✓ 4 tsp canola oil
- ✓ 1 pint blueberries
- ✓ 1/2 cup maple syrup
- ✓ 3 tbsp water
- ✓ 1 tsp lemon juice
- ✓ pinch of salt

Directions

1. Combine all of your dry ingredients in a large mixing bowl and stir to evenly combine.

2. Whisk together all of your wet ingredients in a separate bowl.

3. Make a well in the center of your dry ingredients and begin to slowly pour in the wet ingredients, about a □uarter cup at a time. This will insure that no lumps form when whisking.

4. Continue adding your wet ingredients to the flour base until a smooth batter forms. Let the batter rest for 15 minutes while you preheat your griddle.

5. While the griddle is warming up, make warm maple blueberry compote. Combine blueberries, maply syrup, water, lemon juice, and a pinch salt in a small pot. Stir evenly to mix.

6. Gently heat the pot over medium-low heat until the blueberries begin to pop and release their natural juices. Set aside but keep warm.

7. Once the griddle has been pre-heated to a medium hot temperature, lightly oil the griddle using non-stick spray or a small amount of neutral flavored oil.

8. Ladle the batter on to the griddle, making sure you do not overcrowd your griddle.

9. Allow the pancakes to cook undisturbed until the edges look dry and bubbles come to the surface without breaking. This should take roughly two minutes.

10. Flip the pancakes over and cook on the other side for another two minutes.

11. Keep warm or serve immediately with the warm maple-blueberry compote.

Note: You can keep compote stored in an air-tight container for up to three days.

11. Tofu Turmeric Scramble

Tofu can be intimidating, but this versatile plant protein takes on whatever flavor you give it. With every bite of this savory scramble recipe, you'll feel healthier and invigorated. This breakfast will also help manage your blood sugar levels.

Ingredients

- ✓ 1 8-ounce block of firm or extra-firm tofu, drained
- ✓ 1 tbsp extra virgin olive oil
- ✓ ¼ red onion, chopped
- ✓ 1 green or red bell pepper, chopped

- ✓ 2 cups of fresh spinach, loosely chopped
- ✓ ½ cup sliced button mushrooms
- ✓ ½ tsp each salt and pepper
- ✓ 1 tsp garlic powder
- ✓ ½ tbsp turmeric
- ✓ ¼ cup nutritional yeast

Directions

1. Drain the tofu and squeeze gently to remove extra water. Crumble tofu into a bowl by hand - the smaller the pieces, the better.

2. Prep vegetables and place a large skillet over medium heat. Once ready, add olive oil, onions, and bell peppers. Stir in a pinch of the salt and pepper and cook for about 5 minutes to soften the vegetables. Then add mushrooms and sauté for 2 minutes. Then add tofu. Sauté for about 3 minutes, a little more if the tofu is watery.

3. Add the rest of the salt and pepper, garlic turmeric, and nutritional yeast and mix with a spatula, making sure the spices blend well. Cook for another 5 to 8 minutes until tofu is slightly browned.

4. Add the spinach and cover the pan to steam for 2 minutes. Serve immediately with sides of your choice.

12. Red Pepper, Kale, and Cheddar Frittata

If you want to lose weight but worry you'll have to sacrifice delicious foods, you're in luck. Try adding the vegetables below or mix and match to find your favorite creation.

Ingredients

- ✓ 1 tsp olive oil
- ✓ 5 oz baby kale and spinach
- ✓ 1 red pepper, diced
- ✓ 1/3 cup sliced scallions
- ✓ 12 eggs
- ✓ 3/4 cup milk
- ✓ 1 cup sharp shredded cheddar cheese
- ✓ 1/4 tsp salt
- ✓ 1/4 tsp pepper

Directions

1. Preheat oven to 375°F.

2. Spray an 8 1/2-inch by 12-inch glass or casserole dish with olive oil or nonstick spray.
3. Heat oil in a large frying pan. Add red peppers on low and cook until tender. Add kale and spinach, occasionally stirring until greens are wilted, or for about 3 minutes.
4. Transfer peppers and greens to the dish, spreading evenly. Add sliced scallions.
5. Beat eggs with milk, salt, and pepper. Pour the egg mixture over the pan. Sprinkle cheese on top.
6. Bake about 35-40 minutes or until the mixture is completely set and starting to lightly brown. For additional color, place under broiler for an additional 1 to 3 minutes, watching carefully to make sure the top doesn't burn. Let cool about 5 minutes before cutting.
7. Serve warm or refrigerate for a □uick breakfast during the week. Microwave for 1-2 minutes to reheat.

CHAPTER NINE

RECIPES FOR DASH LUNCH

You should always prep your lunches with fresh vegetables, whole grains, healthy fats, poultry, and fish on The DASH Diet. This plan focuses on foods that help lower your blood pressure to help you live a healthier life. A hearty mid-day meal is the key to keeping your energy up, your mind focused, and your stomach full until dinnertime. Add these recipes into your lunchtime repertoire.

1. Grilled Flat Bread Pizza

Grilling your pizza takes minutes and offers a ton of flavor without extra calories. You can purchase pre-made pizza dough in the dairy section of your local grocery store, make your own dough from scratch, or use pre-made flat breads like Indian naan or Greek pita breads. Once you've grilled the flatbread, load up with your favorite fresh vegetables and spices for a hearty, satsifying lunch or dinner.

Ingredients

- ✓ 1 tbsp olive oil, plus more for topping if desired
- ✓ flatbread dough (use whole grain dough if on the DASH Diet)
- ✓ 1/2 tsp each of dried herbs, red pepper flakes, or other desired spices
- ✓ 1 bunch fresh broccoli, cauliflower, arugula, or other cruciferous vegetables
- ✓ 1 bell pepper, sliced

Directions

1. Heat grill to medium heat and brush a light layer of oil. Cook both sides of flatbread dough until golden brown, about 2 minutes per side.

2. Top flatbread with sliced fresh vegetables and leafy greens. Season with olive oil, salt, pepper, red pepper flakes, or herbs, to taste.

3. Transfer flatbread pizza to oven to finish cooking.

2.Spinach Salad with Walnuts and Strawberries

The combo of tart strawberries, crunchy walnuts, and salty cheese should satisfy every craving! This salad is even more fabulous when tossed with a zero-fat balsamic vinaigrette.

Ingredients

- ✓ 1/2 cup walnuts
- ✓ 4 cups fresh spinach, stems trimmed and roughly chopped
- ✓ 3 tbsp honey
- ✓ 2 tbsp spicy brown mustard
- ✓ 1/4 cup balsamic vinegar
- ✓ 1/4 tsp sea salt
- ✓ 1/4 cup crumbled feta (about 1 oz), optional

Directions

1. Heat the oven to 375°F. Place the walnuts on a rimmed baking sheet and bake until fragrant and toasted, about 8 minutes. Transfer to a plate to cool.

2. Toss the spinach with the strawberries in a large bowl. In a small bowl whisk together the honey, mustard, vinegar, and salt. Drizzle 3/4 of the dressing over the salad and sprinkle the walnuts on top. Serve sprinkled with cheese (if using) and with the remaining dressing on the side.

3. Chicken Vegetable Soup

Chicken soup isn't just for the winter months when you are sick in bed. This protein-packed vegetable chicken soup is perfect to enjoy all year long. You get your protein fix from the chicken and black beans, while getting your vitamin boost from all the vegetables. Add seaweed rich in iodine to increase your energy levels.

Ingredients

- ✓ 2 tbsp olive oil
- ✓ 3 cloves garlic
- ✓ 1 onion
- ✓ 4 cups low-sodium chicken broth
- ✓ 1/2 cup carrot, chopped
- ✓ 1/2 cup parsnip, chopped
- ✓ 2 cups collard green, chopped
- ✓ 1 can black beans, strained
- ✓ 1/2 cup seaweed (optional)

Directions

1. Simmer garlic and onion combined in olive oil.
2. Pour in the chicken broth and the vegetables and turn to a boil. When boiling turn to a simmer.

3. Leave on simmer until vegetables are soft. With 5 minutes left to cook, pour in the strained canned beans and optional seaweed.

4. Avocado Sandwich With Lemon and Cilantro

This sandwich recipe is beneficial in many ways. It's full of naturally good fats, potassium, and vitamin C. With fruit on the side, you'll fulfill both your sweet and salty cravings eating this low-sodium meal.

Ingredients

- ✓ 1 medium Hass avocado
- ✓ 2 slices 100% whole wheat bread
- ✓ 1/2 cup spinach
- ✓ 1/4 cup cilantro
- ✓ 1/2 carrots, sliced
- ✓ 1/4 cucumber, sliced
- ✓ 1/4 cup blueberries
- ✓ 1/4 cup red cherries
- ✓ 1 tbsp lemon juice
- ✓ 1 cup skim milk

Directions

1. Toast bread.

2. Slice avocado into thin strips (or as desired) and place on toast.

3. Slice vegetables and place on toast.

4. Sprinkle with lemon juice and a dash of salt.

5. Prepare the fruit, and enjoy a mixed fruit bowl and skim milk on the side.

5. Creamy Vegetable Lentil Soup

This lentil soup recipe, Packed with fiber, vitamins, and minerals, you can enjoy this dish for lunch, dinner, or anytime in between.

Ingredients

- ✓ 1/4 cup olive oil
- ✓ 1 cup chopped celery
- ✓ 1 cup chopped carrots
- ✓ 1 large white onion, diced
- ✓ 4 cloves garlic, minced
- ✓ 2 cups dry lentils
- ✓ 8 cups water
- ✓ 1 tbsp reduced sodium vegetable bouillon
- ✓ 1 can crushed tomatoes

- ✓ 2 tsp cumin
- ✓ 3 cups spinach, rinsed and roughly chopped
- ✓ 1/4 cup fresh basil chopped or 1 tbsp dried basil
- ✓ 1/2 cup white wine
- ✓ salt to taste
- ✓ ground black pepper to taste

Directions

1. In a large soup pot, heat oil over medium heat. Add carrots, celery and onions and cook, stirring occasionally for about 10 minutes or until the vegetables have softened. Stir in garlic and cook for another minute.
2. Add lentils, water, tomatoes, and cumin. Bring to a boil. Reduce heat to low, and simmer for about one hour or until lentils are tender.
3. When lentils are tender, stir in spinach and basil, and cook until it wilts. Stir in wine, and season to taste with salt and pepper.
4. For a creamy texture, remove about half of soup when cooled and puree in a blender. Add back to pot, garnish with basil, and enjoy!

6. Rocco DiSpirito's Swiss Chard Turkey Salad With Golden Raisins and Capers

Does your go-to salad look a little sad and wilty by the time you pull it out of the fridge during your lunch break? This Swiss chard and turkey salad not only holds up well throughout the day but also provides the fiber, protein, and fat you need to refuel for the afternoon ahead.

Ingredients

- ✓ 1/4 cup chopped golden raisins
- ✓ 2 tbsp water
- ✓ 2 tbsp freshly squeezed lemon juice
- ✓ 2 tbsp chopped capers, plus 1 tsp caper brine
- ✓ 1/4 cup toasted almonds
- ✓ freshly ground black pepper
- ✓ 1/3 cup sliced red onion
- ✓ 1 cup cherry tomatoes
- ✓ 6 cups chopped Swiss chard, stems cut very thin
- ✓ 1 tsp extra-virgin olive oil
- ✓ 6 oz store-roasted skinless turkey breast, shredded
- ✓ 1 chopped avocado (optional)

Directions

1. Combine the raisins in a microwave-safe bowl with the 2 tablespoons water. Cook on high in the microwave until simmering, 1 1/2 to 2 minutes. Remove from the microwave and let stand for 2 minutes.

2. Put the lemon juice, capers and brine, and almonds in a small bowl and season with black pepper. Add the raisins, their soaking liquid, the onion, and the tomatoes and mix well.

3. In a large bowl, combine the Swiss chard, olive oil, and turkey and toss well. Add the mixture from the small bowl and toss together to combine. Spoon the salad onto four salad plates, dividing it e□ually. If using, top the salad with the chopped avocado and serve.

7. Grilled Tofu and Mushroom Burger

If you're craving a burger but don't want the excess fat and calories, give this delicious tofu burger a try. This flavorful and hearty recipe is the perfect healthy lunch or dinner swap.

Ingredients

- ✓ 6 oz firm tofu
- ✓ 4 oz mushrooms
- ✓ 1 medium onion, sliced
- ✓ 1 medium red onion, sliced
- ✓ 2 cloves garlic, diced
- ✓ 2 medium tomatoes, sliced
- ✓ 4 oz cheese (your choice)
- ✓ 1 oz coriander, chopped
- ✓ 1 chilli, finely chopped
- ✓ 1 egg, beaten
- ✓ 1 tbsp flour
- ✓ 4 tbsp canola oil
- ✓ whole wheat hamburger buns
- ✓ salt and pepper, to taste
- ✓ lettuce
- ✓ ketchup
- ✓ mustard

Directions

1. Preheat oven to 275°F.
2. In a pan under medium heat sauté the onions, garlic, chilli, and mushrooms. Set aside to cool.

3. Then in a bowl, add the tofu, mushrooms, coriander, and mash together with a fork.

4. Add the egg and flour and mix into a pliable consistency. Adjust seasonings. Form into patties.

5. In a pan under medium heat fry patties on both sides until golden brown. Place in oven for 5 minutes.

6. Place cheese on the burgers, then turn oven off, and let cheese melt over the burger. Serve and enjoy!

8. Salmon Stuffed Avocado

Salmon is packed with amino acids, protein, vitamins B12 and D. Oily fish is an important part of a healthy diet as their omega-3 fatty acids contribute to healthy brain and heart function. Monosaturated fats are found in avocados and help lower bad LDL cholesterol.

Ingredients

- ✓ 2 avocados, sliced in half
- ✓ 5 oz wild-caught salmon, cooked and cut into small chunks

- ✓ 1/2 cup lettuce, chopped
- ✓ 2 tbsp cilantro, chopped
- ✓ 3 tbsp fresh lemon juice
- ✓ 2 tbsp olive oil
- ✓ 1/2 tsp cumin
- ✓ salt and pepper to taste

Directions

1. Add all ingredients to a bowl and mix gently by hand. Season with salt and pepper as desired.
2. Spoon mixture into each avocado half.

9. "Cobb" Salad

Eating Paleo, or like our Stone-Age ancestors, doesn't mean tearing hunks of meat off a bone. Hit the reset button on your body and eat the diet you were born to eat with these recipes.

Ingredients

- ✓ 2 tbsp extra-virgin olive oil
- ✓ 2 skinless, boneless chicken breast halves (about 1 lb), pounded thin with a meat tenderizer tool
- ✓ 1/4 cup diced leftover roasted turkey breast

- ✓ 1 head romaine lettuce, chopped, rinsed and spun dry
- ✓ 1 small bunch frisée or your choice of lettuce if unavailable, separated, rinsed and spun dry
- ✓ 1 medium avocado, pitted, peeled and sliced
- ✓ 1 medium tomato, seeded (cut in half, then use a spoon to scoop out seeds), and finely chopped
- ✓ 2 large eggs, hard-boiled and sliced into circles
- ✓ 1 tbsp crushed mustard seed
- ✓ 1 tbsp chopped fresh chives
- ✓ 1 tbsp freshly squeezed lemon juice
- ✓ freshly ground black pepper (optional)

Directions

1. Heat the oil in a cast-iron skillet over medium heat. Pat the chicken breasts dry with paper towels and cook for 6 to 8 minutes, flipping halfway. Check with an instant-read thermometer for internal temperature of 160°F. Remove from the heat, place on plate, cover loosely with foil and set aside.

2. Add the diced turkey to the same pan and cook just long enough to crisp, 2 to 3 minutes. Remove from the heat and drain on paper towels.

3. Combine the romaine and frisée and divide equally on two large plates. Slice chicken and place on top. Arrange the turkey, avocado, tomato, and sliced eggs in neat rows on top of the lettuce.

4. In a small bowl, combine the lemon juice, mustard seed and chives. Drizzle on top of salad, followed by pepper, if desired.

10. Veggie Sushi

A simple lunch option, this veggie sushi that Tom Brady and Giselle Bündchen love is perfect for vegans and vegetarians and easy to customize. Made with brown rice instead of white sushi rice, you'll get a serving of whole grains and extra fiber as well!

Ingredients

- ✓ 3 cups brown rice
- ✓ 2 tbsp rice wine vinegar
- ✓ 2 avocados, sliced lengthwise
- ✓ 2 carrots, sliced lengthwise
- ✓ 1 cucumber, sliced lengthwise
- ✓ ponzu sauce, to taste

Directions

1. Cook brown rice according to package instructions. Fold rice wine vinegar into rice. Let rice cool to room temperature.

2. When cool, evenly spread out rice on a bamboo sushi mat with a wooden spoon or dip your hands in a bowl of cool water and spread the rice with your fingers. Layer avocado, carrot, and cucumber slices on top.

3. Use the mat to roll rice and vegetables into a packed roll. Slide mat out and repeat. Slice into 1/2-inch rounds.

11. Cucumber Sandwich

Swap out your bread for cucumbers instead. Cucumbers are wet carbs, meaning they have a high water and fiber content. This perfect combination makes it the best lunch to help beat constipation.

Ingredients

- ✓ 1 cucumbers
- ✓ 2 slices swiss cheese
- ✓ 3 slices of turkey deli meat

Directions

1. Cut the cucmber in half lengthwise. Carve out the inside to make it hollow.

2. Place the meat and cheese inside and enjoy!

12. Chunky Vegetarian Chili With Quinoa

Take this chili for example: the tofu substitute creates a meat-like ☐uality and thickens up the chili so you can still have a hearty meal without the ground beef. This recipe is so tasty that Lisa bets meat-lovers won't even be able to tell the difference. Give this recipe a try and make it in bulk so you can freeze it and save it for when you need a quick, on-the-go lunch or dinner.

Ingredients

- ✓ 2 tbsp extra virgin olive oil
- ✓ 1 large sweet onion, chopped
- ✓ 2 medium carrots, cut into 1/2-inch dice
- ✓ 2 medium celery ribs, cut into 1/2-inch dice
- ✓ 1 jalapeño, seeded and minced
- ✓ 4 garlic cloves, minced
- ✓ 2 tbsp chili powder
- ✓ 2 tsp ground cumin
- ✓ 2 tsp dried oregano

- ✓ 1 28 oz can crushed tomatoes
- ✓ 1 12 oz bottle lager beer
- ✓ 2 tbsp pure maple syrup
- ✓ 1 canned chipotle chile in adobo, minced
- ✓ 1 15 oz can kidney beans, drained and rinsed
- ✓ 1 15 oz can black beans, drained and rinsed
- ✓ fine sea salt and freshly ground black pepper
- ✓ 1 tsp extra virgin olive oil
- ✓ 7 oz extra-firm tofu, pressed and crumbled
- ✓ 1 tsp chili powder
- ✓ 1 tsp ground cumin
- ✓ 1 tsp garlic powder
- ✓ 1/2 tsp fine sea salt
- ✓ 2 cups uinoa (use any color or the rainbow mix)
- ✓ 1 tsp fine sea salt
- ✓ chopped fresh cilantro, for garnish

Directions

1. To make the chili heat two tablespoons of oil in a large pot over medium heat. Add the onion, carrots, celery, jalapeño, and garlic and cook, stirring occassionaly, until the onion is tender, about 10 minutes. Add two tablespoons of chili

powder, two teaspoons of cumin, and oregano, and stir. Add the tomatoes, beet, one cup water, maple syrup, and chipotle and stir well. Bring to a simmer over high heat. Reduce the heat to medium-low and simmer, uncovered, until the vegetables are just tender, about 30 minutes. Stir in the kidney beans and black beans and cook for 10 minutes more.

2. To make the chili tofu heat one teaspoon of oil in a medium skilet over medium heat. Add the tofu and cook, until lightly browned, about three minutes. Combine one teaspoon of chili powder, one teaspoon of cumin, garlic powder, and 1/2 teaspoon of salt in a bowl. Sprinkle the chili mixture over the tofu and stir well. Stir the chili tofu into the chili and cook until it has thickened, about 10 minutes. Season to taste with salt and pepper.

3. To make the quinoa place two cups in a fine-mesh wire sieve and rinse well under cold water (don't skip this step). Drain well. Bring the drained Quinoa, two and a half cups of water, and one teaspoon of salt to a boil in a medium saucepan over high heat. Reduce the heat to

medium-low. Cover and simmer until the quinoa is tender and has absorbed the liquid, 15 to 20 minutes. Remove from the stove and let stand for five minutes. Fluff the quinoa with a fork. Spoon the quinoa into wide soup bowls and top with the chili. Sprinkle with cilantro and serve.

CHAPTER TEN

RECIPES FOR THE DASH APPETIZER

This colorful and tasty Dash Diet appetizer is one of my all time favorites and compliments any meal, it is a delicious Appetizer for any party. The DASH diet has been proved to reduce blood pressure, which can help you live a longer and healthier life. Try these delicious recipes.

1. Grilled pineapple

This Caribbean-style marinade and the heat of the grill give this pineapple dessert a smoky sweetness.

Ingredients

- ✓ For the marinade
- ✓ 2 tablespoons dark honey
- ✓ 1 tablespoon olive oil
- ✓ 1 tablespoon fresh lime juice
- ✓ 1 teaspoon ground cinnamon
- ✓ 1/4 teaspoon ground cloves
- ✓ 1 firm, ripe pineapple

- ✓ 8 wooden skewers, soaked in water for 30 minutes, or metal skewers
- ✓ 1 tablespoon dark rum (optional)
- ✓ 1 tablespoon grated lime zest

Directions

1. Prepare a hot fire in a charcoal grill or heat a gas grill or broiler (grill). Away from the heat source, lightly coat the grill rack or broiler pan with cooking spray. Position the cooking rack 4 to 6 inches from the heat source.

2. To make the marinade, in a small bowl, combine the honey, olive oil, lime juice, cinnamon and cloves and whisk to blend. Set aside.

3. Cut off the crown of leaves and the base of the pineapple. Stand the pineapple upright and, using a large, sharp knife, pare off the skin, cutting downward just below the surface in long, vertical strips and leaving the small brown "eyes" on the fruit. Lay the pineapple on its side. Aligning the knife blade with the diagonal rows of eyes, cut a shallow furrow, following a spiral pattern around the pineapple, to remove all the eyes. Stand the peeled pineapple upright and cut

it in half lengthwise. Place each pineapple half cut-side down and cut it lengthwise into four long wedges; slice away the core. Cut each wedge crosswise into three pieces. Thread the three pineapple pieces onto each skewer.

4. Lightly brush the pineapple with the marinade. Grill or broil, turning once and basting once or twice with the remaining marinade, until tender and golden, about 5 minutes on each side.

5. Remove the pineapple from the skewers and place on a platter or individual serving plates. Brush with the rum, if using, and sprinkle with the lime zest. Serve hot or warm.

2. Gluten-free hummus

This recipe replaces tahini, which sometimes contains gluten, with olive oil. It also calls for sherry vinegar instead of lemon juice.

Ingredients

- ✓ 2/3 cup dried chickpeas (garbanzos), picked over and rinsed, soaked overnight, and drained
- ✓ 3 cups water

- ✓ 2 cloves garlic
- ✓ 1 bay leaf
- ✓ 1/2 teaspoon salt
- ✓ 1 tablespoon olive oil
- ✓ 3/4 cup plus 2 tablespoons sliced green (spring) onion
- ✓ 2 tablespoons sherry vinegar
- ✓ 3 tablespoons chopped fresh cilantro (fresh coriander)
- ✓ 1 teaspoon ground cumin

Directions

1. In a large saucepan over high heat, combine the chickpeas, water, garlic cloves, bay leaf and 1/4 teaspoon of salt. Bring to a boil. Reduce the heat to low, cover partially and simmer until the beans are very tender, 50 to 60 minutes. Drain and discard the bay leaf, reserving the garlic and 1/2 cup of the cooking liquid.

2. In a blender or food processor, combine the chickpeas, cooked garlic, olive oil, 3/4 cup green onion, vinegar, cilantro, cumin and the remaining 1/4 teaspoon salt. Process to puree. Add the reserved cooking liquid, 1 tablespoon at a time,

until the mixture has the consistency of a thick spread.

3. In a small serving bowl, stir together the chickpea mixture and the remaining 2 tablespoons green onion. Serve immediately, or cover and refrigerate until ready to serve. Makes about 1 1/2 cups.

3. Artichoke dip

Serve this dip with raw vegetables or whole-grain crackers.

Ingredients

- ✓ 1 can (15.5 ounces) artichoke hearts in water, drained
- ✓ 4 cups chopped raw spinach
- ✓ 2 cloves garlic, minced
- ✓ 1 teaspoon ground black pepper
- ✓ 1 teaspoon minced fresh thyme (or 1/3 teaspoon dried)
- ✓ 1 tablespoon fresh minced parsley (or 1 teaspoon dried)

- ✓ 1 cup prepared unsalted white beans (or half a 15.5-ounce can unsalted white beans, rinsed and drained)
- ✓ 2 tablespoons grated Parmesan cheese
- ✓ 1/2 cup low-fat sour cream

Directions

1. In a mixing bowl, combine the ingredients. Transfer to an oven-safe glass or ceramic dish and bake at 350 F for 30 minutes. Serve warm.

4. Fruit salsa and sweet chips

This kid-friendly recipe is easy for young cooks to prepare with just a little help from an adult.

Ingredients

For tortilla crisps:

- ✓ 8 whole-wheat fat-free tortillas
- ✓ Cooking spray
- ✓ 1 tablespoon sugar
- ✓ 1/2 tablespoon cinnamon

For fruit salsa:

- ✓ 3 cups diced fresh fruit, such as apples, oranges, kiwi, strawberries, grapes or other fresh fruit
- ✓ 2 tablespoons sugar-free jam, any flavor
- ✓ 1 tablespoon honey or agave nectar
- ✓ 2 tablespoons orange juice

Directions

1. Heat the oven to 350 F. Cut each tortilla into 8 wedges. Lay pieces on two baking sheets. Make sure they aren't overlapping. Spray the tortilla pieces with cooking spray.

2. In a small bowl, combine sugar and cinnamon. Sprinkle evenly over the tortilla wedges. Bake for 10 to 12 minutes or until the pieces are crisp. Place on a cooling rack and let cool.

3. Cut the fruit into cubes. Gently mix the fruit together in a mixing bowl. In another bowl, whisk together jam, honey and orange juice. Pour this over the diced fruit. Mix gently. Cover the bowl with plastic wrap and refrigerate for 2 to 3 hours.

4. Serve as a dip or topping for the cinnamon tortilla chips.

5. Fresh tomato crostini

Crostini is the Italian word for little toasts. These little toasts are topped with a tomato, basil and garlic mixture.

Ingredients

- ✓ 4 plum tomatoes, chopped
- ✓ 1/4 cup minced fresh basil
- ✓ 2 teaspoons olive oil
- ✓ 1 clove garlic, minced
- ✓ Freshly ground pepper
- ✓ 1/4 pound crusty Italian peasant bread, cut into 4 slices and toasted

Directions

1. Combine tomatoes, basil, oil, garlic and pepper in a medium bowl. Cover and let stand 30 minutes. Divide tomato mixture with any juices among the toast. Serve at room temperature.

6. Hummus

Serve this easy Mediterranean spread with warmed whole-wheat pita bread. For a different taste you can substitute white, butter or lima beans for garbanzos and 1 teaspoon toasted ground cumin seeds for the paprika.

Ingredients

- ✓ 2 cans (16 ounces each) reduced-sodium garbanzos, rinsed and drained except for 1/4 cup liquid
- ✓ 1 tablespoon extra-virgin olive oil
- ✓ 1/4 cup lemon juice
- ✓ 2 garlic cloves, minced
- ✓ 1/4 teaspoon cracked black pepper
- ✓ 1/4 teaspoon paprika
- ✓ 3 tablespoons tahini (sesame paste)
- ✓ 2 tablespoons chopped Italian flat-leaf parsley

Note: If you need to follow a gluten-free diet, check the label to make sure the brand of tahini is gluten-free.

Directions

1. In a blender or food processor, add the garbanzos. Process to puree. Combine the olive oil, lemon juice, garlic, pepper, paprika, tahini and parsley. Blend well. Add the reserved liquid, 1 tablespoon at a time until the mixture has the consistency of a thick spread. Serve immediately or cover and refrigerate until ready to serve.

7. Artichoke, spinach and white bean dip

You can puree the beans if you want the dip to have a smoother consistency.

Ingredients

- ✓ 2 cups artichoke hearts
- ✓ 1 tablespoon black pepper
- ✓ 4 cups chopped spinach
- ✓ 1 teaspoon minced dried thyme
- ✓ 2 cloves garlic, minced
- ✓ 1 tablespoon minced fresh parsley
- ✓ 1 cup cooked white beans
- ✓ 2 tablespoons grated parmesan cheese
- ✓ 1/2 cup reduced-fat sour cream

Directions

1. Heat oven to 350 degrees.
2. Mix all ingredients together. Put in a glass or ceramic dish and bake for 30 minutes.
3. Serve with vegetables or whole-grain bread or crackers.

8. Artichokes alla Romana

Globe artichokes look like large, green flower buds. Don't confuse them with Jerusalem artichokes (sunchokes), which are brown and resemble ginger root.

Ingredients

- ✓ 2 cups fresh breadcrumbs, preferably whole-wheat
- ✓ 1 tablespoon olive oil
- ✓ 4 large globe artichokes
- ✓ 2 lemons, halved
- ✓ 1/3 cup grated Parmesan cheese
- ✓ 3 garlic cloves, finely chopped
- ✓ 2 tablespoons finely chopped fresh flat-leaf (Italian) parsley
- ✓ 1 tablespoon grated lemon zest
- ✓ 1/4 teaspoon freshly ground black pepper
- ✓ 1 cup plus 2 to 4 tablespoons low-sodium vegetable or chicken stock
- ✓ 1 cup dry white wine
- ✓ 1 tablespoon minced shallot
- ✓ 1 teaspoon chopped fresh oregano

Directions

1. Heat the oven to 400 F. In a bowl, combine the breadcrumbs and olive oil. Toss to coat. Spread the crumbs in a shallow baking pan and bake, stirring once halfway through, until the crumbs are lightly golden, about 10 minutes. Set aside to cool.

2. Working with 1 artichoke at a time, snap off any tough outer leaves and trim the stem flush with the base. Cut off the top third of the leaves with a serrated knife, and trim off any remaining thorns with scissors. Rub the cut edges with a lemon half to prevent discoloration. Separate the inner leaves and pull out the small leaves from the center. Using a melon baller or spoon, scoop out the fuzzy choke, then squeeze some lemon juice into the cavity. Trim the remaining artichokes in the same manner.

3. In a large bowl, toss the breadcrumbs with the Parmesan, garlic, parsley, lemon zest and pepper. Add the 2 to 4 tablespoons stock, 1 tablespoon at a time, using just enough for the stuffing to begin to stick together in small clumps.

4. Using 2/3 of the stuffing, mound it slightly in the center of the artichokes. Then, starting at the bottom, spread the leaves open and spoon a rounded teaspoon of stuffing near the base of each leaf. (The artichokes can be prepared to this point several hours ahead and kept refrigerated.)
5. In a Dutch oven with a tightfitting lid, combine the 1 cup stock, wine, shallot and oregano. (Note: Don't use cast iron or the cooked artichokes will turn brown.) Bring to a boil, then reduce the heat to low. Arrange the artichokes, stem-end down, in the li□uid in a single layer. Cover and simmer until the outer leaves are tender, about 45 minutes (add water if necessary). Transfer the artichokes to a rack and let cool slightly. Cut each artichoke into □uarters and serve warm.

9. Baked brie envelopes

Prepare this appetizer the day before guests arrive. Keep wrapped in the fridge until ready to bake.

Ingredients

- ✓ 1/2 cup fresh or frozen cranberries
- ✓ 1/2 medium orange, quartered
- ✓ 2 tablespoons sugar
- ✓ 1 cinnamon stick
- ✓ 1 sheet puff pastry dough, cut into 12 1/4-ounce squares
- ✓ 6 ounces Brie cheese, cut into 1/2-ounce cubes
- ✓ 2 tablespoons water
- ✓ 1 egg white

Directions

1. Heat oven to 425 F.
2. Heat a small saute pan to medium-high heat; lightly coat with cooking spray. Reduce heat to low. Place the cranberries, orange, sugar and cinnamon stick in the pan and cook for about 10 minutes, stirring constantly until cranberries are soft and the mixture starts to thicken. Remove from heat and allow to cool. Remove the cinnamon stick and orange quarters.
3. Roll out each square of puff pastry. Place one cube of cheese and 1 teaspoon of cooled cranberry mixture onto each puff pastry square. In a small bowl, combine the water and egg

white. Using a pastry brush, dab a small amount of the egg mixture onto the inside of the puff pastry. Pull one corner of the pastry at a time around the cheese and cranberry mixture like an envelope. Baste the top of the pastry with the egg mixture. Place the envelopes on a baking sheet and bake for 10 to 12 minutes or until golden brown.

10. Basil pesto stuffed mushrooms

This appetizer can be prepared a day in advance. Refrigerate until ready to serve.

Ingredients

- ✓ 20 crimini mushrooms, washed and stems removed

Topping:

- ✓ 1 1/2 cups panko breadcrumbs
- ✓ 1/4 cup melted butter
- ✓ 3 tablespoons chopped fresh parsley

Filling:

- ✓ 2 cups fresh basil leaves
- ✓ 1/4 cup fresh Parmesan cheese
- ✓ 2 tablespoons pumpkin seeds
- ✓ 1 tablespoon olive oil
- ✓ 1 tablespoon fresh garlic
- ✓ 2 teaspoons lemon juice
- ✓ 1/2 teaspoon kosher salt

Directions

1. Heat the oven to 350 F. Line the mushroom caps upside down on a baking sheet.
2. To prepare the topping, in a small bowl, combine the panko, butter and parsley; set aside.

3. To prepare the filling, place the basil, cheese, pumpkin seeds, oil, garlic, lemon juice and salt in a food processor. Process until evenly mixed.

4. Generously stuff the mushroom caps with the basil pesto filling. Sprinkle each mushroom with about 1 teaspoon of panko topping. Gently pat down the topping. Bake for 10 to 15 minutes or until golden brown.

CHAPTER ELEVEN

RECIPES FOR THE DASH DINNER

The DASH diet has been shown to help lower your blood pressure, lose weight, and improve your overall health.

1. Roasted Chicken Thighs with Peppers & Potatoes

My family loves this dish! There's nothing better than oven baked boneless chicken thighs for dinner. It looks and tastes like you fussed, but it is really simple to make. These roasted chicken thighs use healthy olive oil and fresh herbs from my garden.

Ingredients

- ✓ 2 pounds red potatoes (about 6 medium)
- ✓ 2 large sweet red peppers
- ✓ 2 large green peppers
- ✓ 2 medium onions
- ✓ 2 tablespoons olive oil, divided
- ✓ 4 teaspoons minced fresh thyme or 1-1/2 teaspoons dried thyme, divided

- ✓ 3 teaspoons minced fresh rosemary or 1 teaspoon dried rosemary, crushed, divided
- ✓ 8 boneless skinless chicken thighs (about 2 pounds)
- ✓ 1/2 teaspoon salt
- ✓ 1/4 teaspoon pepper

Directions

1) Preheat oven to 450°. Cut potatoes, peppers and onions into 1-in. pieces. Place vegetables in a roasting pan. Drizzle with 1 tablespoon oil; sprinkle with 2 teaspoons each thyme and rosemary and toss to coat. Place chicken over vegetables. Brush chicken with remaining oil; sprinkle with remaining thyme and rosemary. Sprinkle vegetables and chicken with salt and pepper.

2) Roast until a thermometer inserted in chicken reads 170° and vegetables are tender, 35-40 minutes.

2. Test Kitchen Tips

Boneless skinless chicken thighs work well in the slow cooker. The meat shreds easily, yet stays moist due its slightly higher fat content. They're also cheaper than chicken breast, making it ideal for budget-friendly weeknight dinners.

Common olive oil works better for cooking at high heat than virgin or extra-virgin oil. These higher grades have ideal flavor for cold foods, but they smoke at lower temperatures.

Nutrition Facts

1 chicken thigh with 1 cup vegetables: 308 calories, 12g fat (3g saturated fat), 76mg cholesterol, 221mg sodium, 25g carbohydrate (5g sugars, 4g fiber), 24g protein. Diabetic Exchanges: 3 lean meat, 1 starch, 1 vegetable, 1/2 fat.

3. Thai Chicken Pasta Skillet

This gorgeous Bangkok-style pasta has been a faithful standby for many years and always gets loads of praise. For a potluck, we increase it and do it ahead.

Ingredients

- ✓ 6 ounces uncooked whole wheat spaghetti

- ✓ 2 teaspoons canola oil
- ✓ 1 package (10 ounces) fresh sugar snap peas, trimmed and cut diagonally into thin strips
- ✓ 2 cups julienned carrots (about 8 ounces)
- ✓ 2 cups shredded cooked chicken
- ✓ 1 cup Thai peanut sauce
- ✓ 1 medium cucumber, halved lengthwise, seeded and sliced diagonally
- ✓ Chopped fresh cilantro, optional

Directions

1) Cook spaghetti according to package directions; drain.

2) Meanwhile, in a large skillet, heat oil over medium-high heat. Add snap peas and carrots; stir-fry 6-8 minutes or until crisp-tender. Add chicken, peanut sauce and spaghetti; heat through, tossing to combine.

3) Transfer to a serving plate. Top with cucumber and, if desired, cilantro.

Health Tip: Fruits are typically associated with the antioxidant vitamin C, but sugar snap peas are an excellent source as well.

Nutrition Facts

1-1/3 cups: 403 calories, 15g fat (3g saturated fat), 42mg cholesterol, 432mg sodium, 43g carbohydrate (15g sugars, 6g fiber), 25g protein. Diabetic Exchanges: 3 lean meat, 2-1/2 starch, 2 fat, 1 vegetable.

4. Spinach-Orzo Salad with Chickpeas

The first version of this salad was an experiment in mixing together some random ingredients I had on hand. It was a success, and several people at the party asked for the recipe...which meant I had to re-create it! It's healthy, delicious and perfect for warm-weather days.

Ingredients

- ✓ 1 can (14-1/2 ounces) reduced-sodium chicken broth
- ✓ 1-1/2 cups uncooked whole wheat orzo pasta
- ✓ 4 cups fresh baby spinach
- ✓ 2 cups grape tomatoes, halved
- ✓ 2 cans (15 ounces each) chickpeas or garbanzo beans, rinsed and drained
- ✓ 3/4 cup chopped fresh parsley
- ✓ 2 green onions, chopped

DRESSING:

- ✓ 1/4 cup olive oil
- ✓ 3 tablespoons lemon juice
- ✓ 3/4 teaspoon salt
- ✓ 1/4 teaspoon garlic powder
- ✓ 1/4 teaspoon hot pepper sauce
- ✓ 1/4 teaspoon pepper

Directions

1) In a large saucepan, bring broth to a boil. Stir in orzo; return to a boil. Reduce heat; simmer, covered, until al dente, 8-10 minutes.
2) In a large bowl, toss spinach and warm orzo, allowing spinach to wilt slightly. Add tomatoes, chickpeas, parsley and green onions.
3) Whisk together dressing ingredients. Toss with salad.

Nutrition Facts

3/4 cup: 122 calories, 5g fat (1g saturated fat), 0 cholesterol, 259mg sodium, 16g carbohydrate (1g sugars, 4g fiber), 4g protein. Diabetic Exchanges: 1 starch, 1 fat.

5. Peppered Tuna Kabobs

When we barbecue, we like to wow our guests, so dogs and burgers are out! We make tuna skewers topped with salsa—the perfect easy recipe. My five kids like to help me put them together.

Ingredients

- ✓ 1/2 cup frozen corn, thawed
- ✓ 4 green onions, chopped
- ✓ 1 jalapeno pepper, seeded and chopped
- ✓ 2 tablespoons coarsely chopped fresh parsley
- ✓ 2 tablespoons lime juice
- ✓ 1 pound tuna steaks, cut into 1-inch cubes
- ✓ 1 teaspoon coarsely ground pepper
- ✓ 2 large sweet red peppers, cut into 2x1-inch pieces
- ✓ 1 medium mango, peeled and cut into 1-inch cubes

Directions

1) For salsa, in a small bowl, combine the first five ingredients; set aside.

2) Rub tuna with pepper. On four metal or soaked wooden skewers, alternately thread red peppers, tuna and mango.

3) Place skewers on greased grill rack. Cook, covered, over medium heat, turning occasionally, until tuna is slightly pink in center (medium-rare) and peppers are tender, 10-12 minutes. Serve with salsa.

6. Apple-Cherry Pork Medallions

If you think you're too busy to cook a first-class meal, my pork medallions with tangy apple-cherry sauce, rosemary and thyme deliver the goods in a hurry

Ingredients

- ✓ 1 pork tenderloin (1 pound)
- ✓ 1 teaspoon minced fresh rosemary or 1/4 teaspoon dried rosemary, crushed
- ✓ 1 teaspoon minced fresh thyme or 1/4 teaspoon dried thyme
- ✓ 1/2 teaspoon celery salt
- ✓ 1 tablespoon olive oil
- ✓ 1 large apple, sliced

- ✓ 2/3 cup unsweetened apple juice
- ✓ 3 tablespoons dried tart cherries
- ✓ 1 tablespoon honey
- ✓ 1 tablespoon cider vinegar
- ✓ 1 package (8.8 ounces) ready-to-serve brown rice

Directions

1) Cut tenderloin crosswise into 12 slices; sprinkle with rosemary, thyme and celery salt. In a large nonstick skillet, heat oil over medium-high heat. Brown pork on both sides; remove from pan.

2) In same skillet, combine apple, apple juice, cherries, honey and vinegar. Bring to a boil, stirring to loosen browned bits from pan. Reduce heat; simmer, uncovered, 3-4 minutes or just until apple is tender.

3) Return pork to pan, turning to coat with sauce; cook, covered, 3-4 minutes or until pork is tender. Meanwhile, prepare rice according to package directions; serve with pork mixture.

Nutrition Facts

3 ounces cooked pork with 1/3 cup rice and 1/4 cup apple mixture: 349 calories, 9g fat (2g saturated fat), 64mg cholesterol, 179mg sodium, 37g carbohydrate (16g sugars, 4g fiber), 25g protein. Diabetic Exchanges: 3 lean meat, 2-1/2 starch.

7. Asparagus Turkey Stir-Fry

When people try this dish, they ask for the recipe, just as I did when I first tasted it when visiting a friend's home. Tossed in a delicious lemon sauce, this simple skillet dish is sure to satisfy on the busiest of nights. It's a great way to use leftover turkey

Ingredients

- ✓ 2 teaspoons cornstarch
- ✓ 1/4 cup chicken broth
- ✓ 1 tablespoon lemon juice
- ✓ 1 teaspoon soy sauce
- ✓ 1 pound turkey breast tenderloins, cut into 1/2-inch strips
- ✓ 1 garlic clove, minced
- ✓ 2 tablespoons canola oil, divided
- ✓ 1 pound fresh asparagus, trimmed and cut into 1-1/2-inch pieces
- ✓ 1 jar (2 ounces) sliced pimientos, drained

Directions

1) In a small bowl, combine the cornstarch, broth, lemon juice and soy sauce until smooth; set aside. In a large skillet or wok, stir-fry turkey and

garlic in 1 tablespoon oil until meat is no longer pink; remove and keep warm.

2) Stir-fry asparagus in remaining oil until crisp-tender. Add pimientos. Stir broth mixture and add to the pan; cook and stir for 1 minute or until thickened. Return turkey to the pan; heat through.

Nutrition Facts

1-1/4 cups: 205 calories, 9g fat (1g saturated fat), 56mg cholesterol, 204mg sodium, 5g carbohydrate (1g sugars, 1g fiber), 28g protein. Diabetic Exchanges: 3 lean meat, 1-1/2 fat, 1 vegetable.

8. Sweet Onion & Sausage Spaghetti

Sweet onion seasons turkey, adding rich flavor to Mary Relyea's wholesome pasta dish. At home in Canastota, New York, she tosses it together with light cream, basil and tomatoes for a □uick, springy meal in minutes.

Ingredients

- ✓ 6 ounces uncooked whole wheat spaghetti
- ✓ 3/4 pound Italian turkey sausage links, casings removed

✓ 2 teaspoons olive oil

✓ 1 sweet onion, thinly sliced

✓ 1 pint cherry tomatoes, halved

✓ 1/2 cup loosely packed fresh basil leaves, thinly sliced

✓ 1/2 cup half-and-half cream

✓ Shaved Parmesan cheese, optional

Directions

1) Cook spaghetti according to package directions. Meanwhile, in a large nonstick skillet over medium heat, cook sausage in oil for 5 minutes. Add onion; cook 8-10 minutes longer or until meat is no longer pink and onion is tender.

2) Stir in tomatoes and basil; heat through. Add cream; bring to a boil. Drain spaghetti; toss with sausage mixture. Garnish with cheese if desired.

Nutrition Facts

1-1/2 cups: 334 calories, 12g fat (4g saturated fat), 46mg cholesterol, 378mg sodium, 41g carbohydrate (8g sugars, 6g fiber), 17g protein. Diabetic Exchanges: 2-1/2 starch, 2 lean meat, 1 vegetable, 1 fat.

9. Black Bean & Sweet Potato Rice Bowls

With three hungry boys in my house, dinners need to be □uick and filling, and it helps to get in some veggies, too. This one is a favorite because it's hearty and fun to tweak with different ingredients.

Ingredients

✓ 3/4 cup uncooked long grain rice

- ✓ 1/4 teaspoon garlic salt
- ✓ 1-1/2 cups water
- ✓ 3 tablespoons olive oil, divided
- ✓ 1 large sweet potato, peeled and diced
- ✓ 1 medium red onion, finely chopped
- ✓ 4 cups chopped fresh kale (tough stems removed)
- ✓ 1 can (15 ounces) black beans, rinsed and drained
- ✓ 2 tablespoons sweet chili sauce
- ✓ Lime wedges, optional
- ✓ Additional sweet chili sauce, optional

Directions

1) Place rice, garlic salt and water in a large saucepan; bring to a boil. Reduce heat; simmer, covered, until water is absorbed and rice is tender, 15-20 minutes. Remove from heat; let stand 5 minutes.

2) Meanwhile, in a large skillet, heat 2 tablespoons oil over medium-high heat; saute sweet potato 8 minutes. Add onion; cook and stir until potato is tender, 4-6 minutes. Add kale; cook and stir until tender, 3-5 minutes. Stir in beans; heat through.

3) Gently stir 2 tablespoons chili sauce and remaining oil into rice; add to potato mixture. If desired, serve with lime wedges and additional chili sauce.

Health Tip: Sweet potato + kale + black beans = nearly 1/3 of the daily value for fiber per serving!

Nutrition Facts

2 cups: 435 calories, 11g fat (2g saturated fat), 0 cholesterol, 405mg sodium, 74g carbohydrate (15g sugars, 8g fiber), 10g protein.

10. Chicken & Goat Cheese Skillet

Ingredients

- ✓ 1/2 pound boneless skinless chicken breasts, cut into 1-inch pieces
- ✓ 1/4 teaspoon salt
- ✓ 1/8 teaspoon pepper
- ✓ 2 teaspoons olive oil
- ✓ 1 cup cut fresh asparagus (1-inch pieces)
- ✓ 1 garlic clove, minced
- ✓ 3 plum tomatoes, chopped
- ✓ 3 tablespoons 2% milk
- ✓ 2 tablespoons herbed fresh goat cheese, crumbled
- ✓ Hot cooked rice or pasta
- ✓ Additional goat cheese, optional

Directions

1) Toss chicken with salt and pepper. In a large skillet, heat oil over medium-high heat; saute chicken until no longer pink, 4-6 minutes. Remove from pan; keep warm.

2) Add asparagus to skillet; cook and stir over medium-high heat 1 minute. Add garlic; cook and stir 30 seconds. Stir in tomatoes, milk and 2 tablespoons cheese; cook, covered, over medium

heat until cheese begins to melt, 2-3 minutes. Stir in chicken. Serve with rice. If desired, top with additional cheese.

Nutrition Facts

1-1/2 cups chicken mixture: 251 calories, 11g fat (3g saturated fat), 74mg cholesterol, 447mg sodium, 8g carbohydrate (5g sugars, 3g fiber), 29g protein. Diabetic Exchanges: 4 lean meat, 2 fat, 1 vegetable.

11. Bow Ties with Sausage & Asparagus

We love asparagus, so I look for ways to go green. This pasta dish comes together fast on hectic nights and makes wonderful leftovers

Ingredients

- ✓ 3 cups uncooked whole wheat bow tie pasta (about 8 ounces)
- ✓ 1 pound fresh asparagus, trimmed and cut into 1-1/2-inch pieces
- ✓ 1 package (19-1/2 ounces) Italian turkey sausage links, casings removed
- ✓ 1 medium onion, chopped

- ✓ 3 garlic cloves, minced
- ✓ 1/4 cup shredded Parmesan cheese
- ✓ Additional shredded Parmesan cheese, optional

Directions

1) In a 6-qt. stockpot, cook pasta according to package directions, adding asparagus during the last 2-3 minutes of cooking. Drain, reserving 1/2 cup pasta water; return pasta and asparagus to pot.

2) Meanwhile, in a large skillet, cook sausage, onion and garlic over medium heat until no longer pink, 6-8 minutes, breaking sausage into large crumbles. Add to stockpot. Stir in 1/4 cup cheese and reserved pasta water as desired. Serve with additional cheese if desired.

Nutrition Facts

1-1/3 cups: 247 calories, 7g fat (2g saturated fat), 36mg cholesterol, 441mg sodium, 28g carbohydrate (2g sugars, 4g fiber), 17g protein. Diabetic Exchanges: 2 lean meat, 1-1/2 starch, 1 vegetable.

12. Cod and Asparagus Bake

In this bright and lively one-pan dish, green and red veggies back up tender fish, and lemon pulls everything together. You can use grated Parmesan cheese instead of Romano.

Ingredients

- ✓ 4 cod fillets (4 ounces each)
- ✓ 1 pound fresh thin asparagus, trimmed
- ✓ 1 pint cherry tomatoes, halved
- ✓ 2 tablespoons lemon juice
- ✓ 1-1/2 teaspoons grated lemon zest
- ✓ 1/4 cup grated Romano cheese

Directions

1) Preheat oven to 375°. Place cod and asparagus in a 15x10x1-in. baking pan brushed with oil. Add tomatoes, cut sides down. Brush fish with lemon juice; sprinkle with lemon zest. Sprinkle fish and vegetables with Romano cheese. Bake until fish just begins to flake easily with a fork, about 12 minutes.

2) Remove pan from oven; preheat broiler. Broil cod mixture 3-4 in. from heat until vegetables are lightly browned, 2-3 minutes.

Test Kitchen tips

If asparagus isn't in season, fresh green beans make a fine substitute and will cook in about the same amount of time. We tested cod fillets that were about 3/4 in. thick. You'll need to adjust the bake time up or down if your fillets are thicker or thinner.

Nutrition Facts

1 serving: 141 calories, 3g fat (2g saturated fat), 45mg cholesterol, 184mg sodium, 6g carbohydrate (3g sugars, 2g fiber), 23g protein. Diabetic exchanges: 3 lean meat, 1 vegetable.

13. Weeknight Chicken Chop Suey

If you'd like a little extra crunch with this colorful chop suey, serve with chow mein noddles.

Ingredients

- ✓ 4 teaspoons olive oil
- ✓ 1 pound boneless skinless chicken breasts, cut into 1-inch cubes
- ✓ 1/2 teaspoon dried tarragon
- ✓ 1/2 teaspoon dried basil
- ✓ 1/2 teaspoon dried marjoram

- ✓ 1/2 teaspoon grated lemon zest
- ✓ 1-1/2 cups chopped carrots
- ✓ 1 cup unsweetened pineapple tidbits, drained (reserve juice)
- ✓ 1 can (8 ounces) sliced water chestnuts, drained
- ✓ 1 medium tart apple, chopped
- ✓ 1/2 cup chopped onion
- ✓ 1 cup cold water, divided
- ✓ 3 tablespoons unsweetened pineapple juice
- ✓ 3 tablespoons reduced-sodium teriyaki sauce
- ✓ 2 tablespoons cornstarch
- ✓ 3 cups hot cooked brown rice

Directions

1) In a large cast-iron or other heavy skillet, heat oil over medium heat. Add chicken, herbs and lemon zest; saute until lightly browned. Add next 5 ingredients. Stir in 3/4 cup water, pineapple juice and teriyaki sauce; bring to a boil. Reduce heat; simmer, covered, until chicken is no longer pink and the carrots are tender, 10-15 minutes.

2) Combine cornstarch and remaining water. Gradually stir into chicken mixture. Bring to a

boil; cook and stir until thickened, about 2 minutes. Serve with rice.

Test Kitchen tips

While chop suey is a well-known dish, we're not entirely sure where it came from. Stories abound. Did a visiting chef from China bring us this dish? Was it created to serve miners during the California gold rush? Whatever the origin, it's really a delicious and □uick weeknight meal.

This dish is a great way to eat more veggies! Toss in whatever you have on hand, like green pepper, bok choy, broccoli or kale.

Drizzle on some Sriracha for a spicy kick.

Nutrition Facts

1 cup chop suey with 1/2 cup rice: 330 calories, 6g fat (1g saturated fat), 42mg cholesterol, 227mg sodium, 50g carbohydrate (14g sugars, 5g fiber), 20g protein. Diabetic exchanges: 3 vegetable, 3 lean meat, 1 fruit, 1 fat.

14. Beef and Blue Cheese Penne with Pesto

Uni□ue and simple to prepare, this delicious pasta dish is filled with fresh flavors, and it's as healthy as it is hearty. Best of all, it takes just 30 minutes to set this meal on the table

Ingredients

- ✓ 2 cups uncooked whole wheat penne pasta
- ✓ 2 beef tenderloin steaks (6 ounces each)
- ✓ 1/4 teaspoon salt
- ✓ 1/4 teaspoon pepper
- ✓ 5 ounces fresh baby spinach (about 6 cups), coarsely chopped
- ✓ 2 cups grape tomatoes, halved
- ✓ 1/3 cup prepared pesto
- ✓ 1/4 cup chopped walnuts
- ✓ 1/4 cup crumbled Gorgonzola cheese

Directions

1) Cook pasta according to package directions.
2) Meanwhile, sprinkle steaks with salt and pepper. Grill steaks, covered, over medium heat or broil 4 in. from heat 5-7 minutes on each side or until meat reaches desired doneness (for medium-

rare, a thermometer should read 135°; medium, 140°; medium-well, 145°).

3) Drain pasta; transfer to a large bowl. Add spinach, tomatoes, pesto and walnuts; toss to coat. Cut steak into thin slices. Serve pasta mixture with beef; sprinkle with cheese.

Nutrition Facts

1 serving: 532 calories, 22g fat (6g saturated fat), 50mg cholesterol, 434mg sodium, 49g carbohydrate (3g sugars, 9g fiber), 35g protein.

15. Stir-Fry Rice Bowl

My meatless version of Korean bibimbap is tasty, pretty and easy to tweak for different spice levels.

Ingredients

- ✓ 1 tablespoon canola oil
- ✓ 2 medium carrots, julienned
- ✓ 1 medium zucchini, julienned
- ✓ 1/2 cup sliced baby portobello mushrooms
- ✓ 1 cup bean sprouts
- ✓ 1 cup fresh baby spinach
- ✓ 1 tablespoon water

- ✓ 1 tablespoon reduced-sodium soy sauce
- ✓ 1 tablespoon chili garlic sauce
- ✓ 4 large eggs
- ✓ 3 cups hot cooked brown rice
- ✓ 1 teaspoon sesame oil

Directions

1) In a large skillet, heat canola oil over medium-high heat. Add carrots, zucchini and mushrooms; cook and stir 3-5 minutes or until carrots are crisp-tender. Add bean sprouts, spinach, water, soy sauce and chili sauce; cook and stir just until spinach is wilted. Remove from heat; keep warm.

2) Place 2-3 in. of water in a large skillet with high sides. Bring to a boil; adjust heat to maintain a gentle simmer. Break cold eggs, 1 at a time, into a small bowl; holding bowl close to surface of water, slip egg into water.

3) Cook, uncovered, 3-5 minutes or until whites are completely set and yolks begin to thicken but are not hard. Using a slotted spoon, lift eggs out of water.

4) Serve rice in bowls; top with vegetables. Drizzle with sesame oil. Top each serving with a poached egg.

Nutrition Facts

1 serving: 305 calories, 11g fat (2g saturated fat), 186mg cholesterol, 364mg sodium, 40g carbohydrate (4g sugars, 4g fiber), 12g protein. Diabetic Exchanges: 2 starch, 1 medium-fat meat, 1 vegetable, 1 fat.

16. Green Curry Salmon with Green Beans

Like a lot of people here in the beautiful Pacific Northwest, my boyfriend, Michael, loves to fish. When we have an abundance of fresh salmon on hand, this is one way we cook it.

Ingredients

- ✓ 4 salmon fillets (4 ounces each)
- ✓ 1 cup light coconut milk
- ✓ 2 tablespoons green curry paste
- ✓ 1 cup uncooked instant brown rice
- ✓ 1 cup reduced-sodium chicken broth
- ✓ 1/8 teaspoon pepper
- ✓ 3/4 pound fresh green beans, trimmed
- ✓ 1 teaspoon sesame oil
- ✓ 1 teaspoon sesame seeds, toasted
- ✓ Lime wedges

Directions

1) Preheat oven to 400°. Place salmon in an 8-in. square baking dish. Whisk together coconut milk and curry paste; pour over salmon. Bake, uncovered, until fish just begins to flake easily with a fork, 15-20 minutes.

2) Meanwhile, in a small saucepan, combine rice, broth and pepper; bring to a boil. Reduce heat; simmer, covered, 5 minutes. Remove from heat; let stand 5 minutes.

3) In a large saucepan, place steamer basket over 1 in. of water. Place green beans in basket; bring

water to a boil. Reduce heat to maintain a simmer; steam, covered, until beans are crisp-tender, 7-10 minutes. Toss with sesame oil and sesame seeds.

4) Serve salmon with rice, beans and lime wedges. Spoon coconut sauce over the salmon.

Note: This recipe was tested with Thai Kitchen Green Curry Paste. Health Tip: This nutrition-packed complete meal is gluten-free, heart-smart and diabetic-friendly.

Nutrition Facts

1 serving: 366 calories, 17g fat (5g saturated fat), 57mg cholesterol, 340mg sodium, 29g carbohydrate (5g sugars, 4g fiber), 24g protein. Diabetic Exchanges: 3 lean meat, 2 starch, 1 fat.

17. Chicken Veggie Packets

People think I went to a lot of trouble when I serve these packets. Individual aluminum foil pouches hold the juices in during baking to keep the herbed chicken moist and tender. The foil saves time and makes cleanup a breeze.

Ingredients

- ✓ 4 boneless skinless chicken breast halves (4 ounces each)
- ✓ 1/2 pound sliced fresh mushrooms
- ✓ 1-1/2 cups fresh baby carrots
- ✓ 1 cup pearl onions
- ✓ 1/2 cup julienned sweet red pepper
- ✓ 1/4 teaspoon pepper
- ✓ 3 teaspoons minced fresh thyme
- ✓ 1/2 teaspoon salt, optional
- ✓ Lemon wedges, optional

Directions

1) Flatten chicken breasts to 1/2-in. thickness; place each on a piece of heavy-duty foil (about 12 in. square). Layer the mushrooms, carrots, onions and red pepper over chicken; sprinkle with pepper, thyme and salt if desired.

2) Fold foil around chicken and vegetables and seal tightly. Place on a baking sheet. Bake at 375° for 30 minutes or until chicken juices run clear. If desired, serve with lemon wedges.

Nutrition Facts

1 serving: 175 calories, 3g fat (1g saturated fat), 63mg cholesterol, 100mg sodium, 11g carbohydrate (6g sugars, 2g fiber), 25g protein. Diabetic exchanges: 3 lean meat, 2 vegetable.

18. Butternut Turkey Soup

Although chock-full of lots of nutritious vegetables and turkey, this soup is also light and luscious.

Ingredients

- ✓ 3 shallots, thinly sliced
- ✓ 1 teaspoon olive oil
- ✓ 3 cups reduced-sodium chicken broth
- ✓ 3 cups cubed peeled butternut squash (3/4-inch cubes)
- ✓ 2 medium red potatoes, cut into 1/2-inch cubes
- ✓ 1-1/2 cups water
- ✓ 2 teaspoons minced fresh thyme
- ✓ 1/2 teaspoon pepper
- ✓ 2 whole cloves
- ✓ 3 cups cubed cooked turkey breast

Directions

1) In a large saucepan coated with cooking spray, cook shallots in oil over medium heat until tender. Stir in the broth, squash, potatoes, water, thyme and pepper.

2) Place cloves on a double thickness of cheesecloth; bring up corners of cloth and tie with string to form a bag. Stir into soup. Bring to a boil. Reduce heat; cover and simmer for 10-15 minutes or until vegetables are tender. Stir in turkey; heat through. Discard spice bag.

Nutrition Facts

1-1/3 cups: 192 calories, 2g fat (0 saturated fat), 60mg cholesterol, 332mg sodium, 20g carbohydrate (3g sugars, 3g fiber), 25g protein. Diabetic Exchanges: 3 lean meat, 1 starch.

19. Chicken with Celery Root Puree

Celeriac, or celery root, is a root veggie that combines well with other seasonal ingredients and adds nice texture and flavor to this puree

Ingredients

- ✓ 4 boneless skinless chicken breast halves (6 ounces each)
- ✓ 1/2 teaspoon pepper
- ✓ 1/4 teaspoon salt
- ✓ 3 teaspoons canola oil, divided
- ✓ 1 large celery root, peeled and chopped (about 3 cups)
- ✓ 2 cups chopped peeled butternut squash
- ✓ 1 small onion, chopped
- ✓ 2 garlic cloves, minced
- ✓ 2/3 cup unsweetened apple juice

Directions

1) Sprinkle chicken with pepper and salt. In a large nonstick skillet coated with cooking spray, heat 2 teaspoons oil over medium heat. Brown chicken on both sides. Remove chicken from pan.

2) In same pan, heat remaining oil over medium-high heat. Add celery root, squash and onion;

cook and stir until s□uash is crisp-tender. Add garlic; cook 1 minute longer.

3) Return chicken to pan; add apple juice. Bring to a boil. Reduce heat; simmer, covered, 12-15 minutes or until a thermometer inserted in chicken reads 165°.

4) Remove chicken; keep warm. Cool vegetable mixture slightly. Process in a food processor until smooth. Return to pan and heat through. Serve with chicken.

Nutrition Facts

1 chicken breast half with 2/3 cup puree: 328 calories, 8g fat (1g saturated fat), 94mg cholesterol, 348mg sodium, 28g carbohydrate (10g sugars, 5g fiber), 37g protein. Diabetic Exchanges: 5 lean meat, 2 starch, 1/2 fat.

20. Pepper Ricotta Primavera

Garlic, peppers and herbs top creamy ricotta cheese in this meatless skillet meal you can make in just 20 minutes.

Ingredients

- ✓ 1 cup part-skim ricotta cheese
- ✓ 1/2 cup fat-free milk
- ✓ 4 teaspoons olive oil
- ✓ 1 garlic clove, minced
- ✓ 1/2 teaspoon crushed red pepper flakes
- ✓ 1 medium green pepper, julienned
- ✓ 1 medium sweet red pepper, julienned
- ✓ 1 medium sweet yellow pepper, julienned
- ✓ 1 medium zucchini, sliced
- ✓ 1 cup frozen peas, thawed
- ✓ 1/4 teaspoon dried oregano
- ✓ 1/4 teaspoon dried basil
- ✓ 6 ounces fettuccine, cooked and drained

Directions

1) Whisk together ricotta cheese and milk; set aside. In a large skillet, heat oil over medium heat. Add garlic and pepper flakes; saute 1 minute. Add next 7 ingredients. Cook and stir over medium heat until vegetables are crisp-tender, about 5 minutes.

2) Add cheese mixture to fettuccine; top with vegetables. Toss to coat. Serve immediately.

Test Kitchen tips

- This is a milder flavored dish with a spicy kick. To punch up the flavor use fresh herbs in place of dried.
- Sprinkle with parmesan cheese before serving.

Nutrition Facts

1 cup: 229 calories, 7g fat (3g saturated fat), 13mg cholesterol, 88mg sodium, 31g carbohydrate (6g sugars, 4g fiber), 11g protein. Diabetic Exchanges: 2 starch, 1 medium-fat meat, 1/2 fat.

CHAPTER TWELVE

RECIPES FOR DESSERT DASH

You don't have to give up snacks and dessert to be healthy. On The DASH Diet you are allowed to indulge in both snacks and dessert. But since this diet focuses on foods that help lower your blood pressure to help you live a healthier life, you shouldn't have anything processed or anything that contains a large amount of sugar. Start living your best life today with these healthier options for snacks and desserts.

1. Baked Hard-Boiled Eggs

Baking your eggs is just another way to make hard boiled eggs that seems easier for most people – and they turn out perfect every time! You can either put the eggs directly on the rack or put them in a muffin tin, although we recommend the tin to keep the eggs in place. Bake times range from 20 minutes to 30 minutes depending on your oven, so take one out at 20 minutes and see how close to being done it is.

Ingredients

- ✓ 12 eggs
- ✓ cold water

Directions

1. Place a dozen eggs (or however many you want) in a mini or regular muffin tin.
2. Preheat the oven to 325°, then put the eggs in and bake for 30 minutes.
3. Remove from the oven and instantly immerse in cold water for 10 minutes.
4. For easiest peeling, remove the shells right away, otherwise refrigerate until needed.

2. Rocco DiSpirito's Turkey Jerky

Jerky is a great, high-protein snack, but most store-bought jerky is packed with nitrates which are unhealthy and have been shown to cause cancer. Eliminate the worry and the calories by making your own turkey jerky with this quick and easy recipe.

Ingredients

- ✓ 1 1/2 oz extra lean ground turkey
- ✓ 1/8 tsp salt
- ✓ 1/2 tsp sugar replacement
- ✓ 1/4 tsp smoked paprika
- ✓ 1/8 tsp blackening spice

Directions

1. Add the turkey, spices, and salt to a mixing bowl and mix everything together until a smooth paste forms: you really need to work this hard it takes about two minutes.
2. Lay out plastic wrap on the counter that's at least 12 inches long. Place the paste in the middle and place another piece of plastic wrap over the top. Roll the paste with a rolling pin into a thin sheet about 1/8 inch thick, seven inches long and two inches wide.
3. Cut the wrap lengthwise to make strips. Remove the top layer of plastic and flip the strips onto a microwave safe flat plate. Peel off the other layer of plastic wrap.
4. Cook on high for one minute, flip and cook for 30 seconds. Add a paper towel under the jerky and cook until dried and almost crisp, about another

20 seconds. Remove and place on a plate with paper towels.

5. Repeat steps with the other sheets, let cool and serve. Tip: If you like leathery jerky instead of crispy, cook strips 30 seconds less.

3. Protein Energy Bites

Keep these little bites in your freezer for a □uick burst of energy when you feel tired or are simply looking for a sweet treat. The nuts, seeds, and other healthy ingredients in this recipe are guaranteed to boost your mood and make for a filling snack.

Ingredients

- ✓ 1 cup cashews (soaked for a few hours in water, drained and rinsed)
- ✓ 1/4 cup raisins
- ✓ 1 tbsp chia seeds
- ✓ 1/4 cup sunflower seeds
- ✓ 2 tsp vanilla extract
- ✓ 1 tbsp coconut oil, melted
- ✓ 4 dates (softened in some hot water for 10 minutes, then roughly chopped)
- ✓ pinch sea salt
- ✓ 1/3 cup dried milk powder
- ✓ cocoa powder or finely shredded unsweetened coconut for coating (optional)

Directions

1. Purée all ingredients in a food processor until smooth. Transfer to a bowl and refrigerate for about an hour.

2. Once cold and firm, portion out mixture with a teaspoon or very small scoop and roll into balls (about 3/4 inch in diameter). If you want, you can then roll them in some cocoa powder or shredded coconut for a coating.

3. Store in a bag or airtight container in the freezer.

4. **Debbie Matenopoulos' Savory Summer Fruit Salad**

Ingredients

- ✓ 3-4 cups ripe watermelon, cut into 2-inch cubes
- ✓ 2 fresh, ripe peaches, halved, pitted, and thinly sliced
- ✓ 1/2 lb brine-packed Greek feta, drained and crumbled
- ✓ 1/2 seedless English cucumber, peeled and diced
- ✓ 2 tbsp chiffonade-cut fresh mint leaves
- ✓ 2-3 tbsp honey, to taste

Directions

1. Serves 4.

2. Combine all of the ingredients except the honey in a large salad bowl. Drizzle the honey over the top, toss together, and serve immediately.

5. Huevo Ranchero

Ingredients

- ✓ 1/2 cup black beans (or fat-free refried black beans)
- ✓ dash cumin, if desired
- ✓ 1/2 thin slice red onion
- ✓ 1/2 oz. shredded reduced-fat cheese
- ✓ 1 egg
- ✓ 2 Tbsp. sugar-free salsa
- ✓ 2 Tbsp. guacamole (homemade without out salt, will reduce sodium)

Directions

1) Poach egg in simmering water. While egg is poaching, put beans in a microwave-safe bowl, and mash slightly with a dash of cumin, if desired. Top with onion and cheese, and

microwave for about 30-45 seconds, until cheese is melted. Top with egg and then salsa, and put guacamole on side.

6. Not-Too-Spicy Glazed Nuts

Spice up your average snack by glazing nuts! This recipe contains heart-healthy fats, fibers, and oils and keeps your blood sugar in check. Customize it by switching up the nut assortment to your choosing.

Ingredients

- 1 tbsp extra-virgin olive oil
- 1 tbsp pure maple syrup
- 1 garlic clove, minced
- 1 tsp cumin seeds
- 1 tsp nigella seeds
- 1 tsp oregano, dried
- 1/8 tsp cayenne pepper
- 2 1/2 cups unsalted assorted nuts
- 1/2 tsp fine sea salt
- 1/2 cup pecan halves
- 1/2 cup walnut halves
- 1/2 cup skinned hazelnuts
- 1/2 cup shelled pistachios
- 1/2 cup natural almonds

Directions

1. Position a rack in the center of the oven and preheat the oven to 350°F.

2. In a large bowl, mix the oil, maple syrup, garlic, cumin and nigella seeds, oregano, and cayenne. Add the nuts and mix well to coat the nuts. Sprinkle and toss the nuts with the salt. Spread the nuts on a large rimmed baking sheet.

3. Bake, stirring occasionally to bring the nuts that cook more □uickly around the edges into the center, until the nuts are lightly toasted and glazed, about 20 minutes. Let cool on the baking sheet. Break apart the nuts.

4. The nuts can be stored in an airtight container at room temperature for up to 10 days.

7. **Microwaved Sweet Potato Chips**

When feeling stressed or anxious, chips are one of the ways to release that tension. Instead of reaching for the sodium-filled and greasy chips that you usually would, give these sweet potato chips a try. They are as crunchy as your regular option, fast to make, and much healthier for you.

Ingredients

✓ 2 sweet potatoes

✓ dash olive oil

✓ pinch sea salt

Directions

1. Slice the sweet potatoes very thin.
2. Drizzle them with olive oil and sprinkle over with sea salt.
3. Place them in the microwave and set on high until some of the pieces turn brown, about 2-3 minutes.
4. Flip them over and microwave again.
5. Eat them by themselves

8. Baked Apple Stuffed With Blue Cheese, Walnuts, and Dates

If you like gourmet desserts, then this recipe is definitely for you. The combination of blue cheese, walnuts, dates, and apples is truly a sweet and savory delight. Make one for yourself or several for the family with this □uick and easy microwaveable recipe.

Ingredients

✓ 1 tsp blue cheese

- ✓ 1 tbsp roughly chopped walnuts
- ✓ 1 pitted date
- ✓ 1 large apple

Directions

1. Cut off the top of the apple and core it.
2. Mix blue cheese with the chopped nuts and fill the date with the mixture.
3. Insert the stuffed date into the cored apple. Place on a microwave-safe dish and cook for four to five minutes until apple is soft.

9. Black Bean Brownies

These black bean brownies will have mouths watering and then jaws dropping. With this recipe, there's no need to sacrifice taste come dessert. It's all baked into the mix.

Ingredients

- ✓ 1 1/2 cups black beans, drained, rinsed (1 15-ounce can)
- ✓ 2 tbsp cocoa powder
- ✓ 1/2 cup □uick oats

- ✓ 1/4 tsp salt
- ✓ 1/3 cup pure maple syrup or agave (for non-vegans, honey is fine)
- ✓ 2 tbsp sugar
- ✓ 1/4 cup coconut or vegetable oil
- ✓ 2 tsp pure vanilla extract
- ✓ 1/2 tsp baking powder
- ✓ 1/2-2/3 cup chocolate chips

Directions

1. Preheat oven to 350°F.

2. Pulse all ingredients, except chocoloate chips, in a food processor until completely smooth. Really blend well. (For texture, a food processor works best. A blender is fine if necessary.)

3. Stir in chocolate chips and pour into a greased 8×8 pan. Optional: Sprinkle extra chocolate chips over the top.

4. Cook for 15–18 minutes. Let cool at least 10 minutes before trying to cut (yields about 9–12 squares). If they look a bit undercooked, you can place them in the fridge overnight and they will firm up.

10. Crown Jewel Pie

This is a slightly modified Hungry Girl recipe. Prep time is about 6-7 hours due to Jell-o setting time.

Ingredients

- ✓ One 4-serving package Jell-O Sugar Free Orange Gelatin dessert mix
- ✓ One 4-serving package Jell-O Sugar Free Lime Gelatin dessert mix
- ✓ One 4-serving package Jell-O Sugar Free Strawberry Banana Gelatin dessert mix
- ✓ One 4-serving package Jell-O Sugar Free Strawberry Gelatin dessert mix
- ✓ Half an 8-ounce container Cool Whip Free, thawed
- ✓ 10 Honey maid square crackers (2-1/2" s☐uares)

Directions

1. In a medium bowl, combine Orange mix with 1 cup boiling water, and stir for at least 2 minutes (until completely dissolved). Then add 1/2 cup cold water, and transfer mixture to a s☐uare or rectangular medium container. Place container

in the fridge. Repeat this process with other Jell-o flavors (transferring each to its own container). Refrigerate until firm (about 4 hours or overnight).

2. Once gelatins are firm, slide a knife along the sides of each to release them from the containers. Cut each into half-inch cubes, and place cubes in the fridge.

3. In a large bowl, combine Strawberry mix with 1 cup boiling water, and stir for at least 2 minutes (until completely dissolved). Then add 1/2 cup cold water, and place bowl in the fridge. Refrigerate for about 45 minutes (until slightly thickened but still mixable).

4. Meanwhile, arrange 10 crackers to line bottom of 9 inch pie pan or rectangular pan. (You may have to break them in half for a snuggly fit)

5. Once the Strawberry gelatin has thickened slightly, vigorously stir in the Cool Whip until completely blended (use a whisk if you've got one). Very gently stir cubes into the Cool Whip/Jell-O mixture. Give the sides of the cake pan containing the crust a light mist with nonstick spray. Then pour the contents of the

bowl into the pan. Refrigerate until firm (at least 3 hours).

6. Cut pie into 8 slices, and ENJOY!

CHAPTER THIRTEEN

SUSTAINING THE WEIGHT LOST

More often than not when we embark on a diet we tend to have difficulties in maintaining weight after we've initially lost it. So have you ever found that you put on weight easily or end up back at s□uare one within a few weeks of ending your diet? In f the answer is 'yes' then reading this guide will help you understand why this seems to happen more often than not.

Consider this. When dieting, if you maintain your weight loss for a long period of time this will greatly decrease the chances of you yo-yo dieting and constantly returning to square one. If you want to know why this happens then read on; not only will it help you understand how your body generally reacts to weight loss it will also help you put an action plan into place, to ensure you maintain the said weight loss.

Your idea of your ideal weight Vs Your body's idea of your ideal weight

Have you ever wondered how a certain person in the office can get away with eating chocolate and crisps all the time but never ever seem to put on weight? Most people will say "it's not fair she can eat what she wants and not put on an ounce, she must have super high metabolic rate". However, research, which has been undertaken has blown this theory out of the water.

It suggests that one of the main reasons why some people can eat what they want and not gain weight, while others can't, is because the brain has an idea of what your minimum weight should be and will work overtime to try and regulate your body to stay at that weight. Therefore it suggests that the slim person's body will see to it that their weight doesn't deviate too much form what it considers to be 'normal'.

On the other hand if a person, who's weighed 12 stones for most of their adult life suddenly embarks on a weight loss regime and manages to get down to 10 stones. Then that person will find that their body is fighting to get back to 12 stones.

One of the theories behind the difficulty in maintaining weight is the fact that some of us of have inherited an inbuilt bodily mechanism, which has been passed down through the generations. The mechanism - during times of famine - is what kept a lot of people alive. It is said that the people who carried more fat, would be more likely to survive a famine (which happened often in the past). Nowadays - because food is readily available and is relatively in-expensive this bodily function has become somewhat obsolete, pretty much like our need for the sixth sense.

Maintaining weight - How do I change my body's idea of my ideal weight?

The best way to change your body's idea of its ideal weight is to shock it or trick it into thinking that you're normal weight is lower than it first thought. One of the best things you can do is to ensure that you don't lose weight too quickly if you're dieting, because if you do, when you decide to treat yourself, by, let's say eating a Chinese take-away your body will see it as the perfect opportunity to adjust your weight to what it sees as ideal.

Secondly, once you get down to what you consider to be your ideal weight make sure you maintain it, the longer you do (at least 3 months is recommended) the more likely it is, that your body will see your new weight as 'normal' and ensure that it regulates itself in and around that weight. Therefore if you decide to treat yourself every now and again, your body won't punish you too much and more importantly it will vastly reduce the chances of you yo-yo dieting.

The bottom line is just make sure that once you get down to a weight you're happy with, you don't change your mindset right away. Be disciplined, you'll benefit for years to come.

How to Maintain Weight After Losing Weight

You used to be very overweight, through the past few months you have worked extremely hard to get yourself back on the right track and you like where your healthy lifestyle is right now. Many a times a situation occurs when people lose a big amount of weight only to start going back to their unhealthy ways and seeing that their weight is right where it was a year ago despite all their hard work. The schedule or process you have followed to get to your current acceptable weight should not be forgotten now that you are satisfied. You have to learn to maintain your weight loss. In this article you will learn how you can maintain the healthy lifestyle you have worked so hard for, especially with the help of the best diet around Calorie Shifting Diet.

> **Keep up with the great diet you have been using thus far.**

When you get to a point where your body is looking great, you have to remember to keep a calorie based diet where you watching the number of calorie intake. One of the very best diets currently out there to maintain your weight loss is the Calorie Shifting Diet. You need to provide your body with a lot of antioxidants so drink lots of vitamin C, as naturally as you can. You need to be on a very balanced diet, because a healthy brain keeps a healthy body on track.

> **Stay in tune with your workout activities.**

I know you have been working your bottom off in the gym to lose the weight you currently have so reading this you'll probably roll your eyes. But don't worry; I have good news for you. Hard work always pays off, and in this case you are allowed to slightly take a back seat as to how hard you need to exercise. Throughout your weight loss plan however long you were working out for per day you are now allowed to cut that time in half, while still keeping up with the intensity you had previously.

> ➢ **Don't fall in to the lazy trap now and lose all the effort you have put in to your body.**

With all the information provided in the article you should be well on your way to maintaining your new great shaped life. Don't give up on the healthy foods no matter how tempting those chili cheese fries may look, and cut your workout time in half while using the same fire as if you were 50 pounds overweight. I wish you good luck in maintaining the life that has been destined for you.

If you are like me, who doesn't have time and patience to lose weight through exercise and dieting then the only other natural and healthy option to lose weight fast is through 100% natural weight loss remedies.

How to Maintain Weight Loss For Life

If you have worked hard to lose weight, you will want to enjoy your new healthy weight for the rest of your life. Here are ten tips for achieving lifelong weight maintenance:

1. Monitor Your Weight

Weigh yourself once a week (do not weigh yourself too often it is natural for your weight to fluctuate daily). Use your bathroom scales, or find a pair of pants that are comfortable at your goal weight and identify if they get significantly tighter or looser.

It is normal for your weight to fluctuate by 1-2 kilograms, but if you notice your weight increasing on two or more consecutive weeks try one (or a combination) of the following three actions:

1) Decrease your calorie intake
2) Increase the duration and / or frequency of your exercise sessions
3) Change any areas of your lifestyle, behaviour or environment that could be hindering your weight management efforts.

You should set an upper and a lower limit on your weight (a Dietitian can help you set appropriate limits). If you hit your upper or lower limit, seek professional help from a Dietitian as soon as possible. And do not procrastinate for too long - it is much easier to reverse a

1-2kg weight gain than it is to reverse a 5-7kg weight gain!

2. Monitor Your Eating Patterns

It is important that you maintain a consistent eating pattern for the rest of your life - do not change it too drastically on weekends or when you go away on holidays.

Documenting what you eat is a great habit. By keeping a food diary you can ensure that you are eating the right amounts of food from each of the five food groups and check that you are eating regularly (that means not skipping any meals).

3. Exercise

Hopefully you engaged in regular exercise while you were losing weight. To maintain your weight you need to exercise at a moderate intensity (a rate at which your heart rate is elevated but you can still carry out a conversation) for at least 150 minutes per week. A great way to achieve this is to walk for 30 minutes on five days of every week. For the fitter members of the audience, you can try vigorous cardiovascular exercise such as jogging for 20 minutes a day on three days of every week.

If you want to change the shape of your body or strengthen your muscles, try resistance training. Resistance training is performing exercise against an opposing force such as water, free weights, weight machines, a theraband, a fit ball or even your own body weight. Resistance training offers many benefits: it increases the proportion of lean body tissue (muscle) in your body contributing to a higher metabolic rate. Plus it improves your posture, flexibility and strength. If you are interested in starting a resistance training program, it is best to have a program designed by an Exercise Physiologist or a personal trainer.

4. Continue to Set Goals

The goal of weight loss is change, whereas the goal of weight maintenance is no change. It can be harder to eat well and exercise when you do not see results for the effort you are putting in. To account for this, try setting other life goals that are better enjoyed at a lower weight (e.g. joining a community fun walk or going travelling).

5. Reward Yourself

When you were losing weight you were probably enjoying the associated rewards the complements from other people, the excitement of fitting into smaller clothes and the joy of jumping onto the scales and seeing a smaller number. So you will need a new set of rewards for maintaining your weight. Perhaps you can treat yourself to a massage, buy a book or have a manicure of pedicure at the end of every month. Continue these rewards for at least the first few years after weight loss.

6. Enlist Support

While you were losing weight you probably received encouragement from family, friends and health professionals. Weight maintenance can be just as difficult as weight loss at times - and it can be a more isolated process. But it does not have to be that way. Tell the important people in your life that maintaining your healthy weight is important to you, and that you would like their support and encouragement for the long term.

7. Remain Vigilant

It is easy to get complacent when you achieve your weight loss goal. People sometimes fall into the trap of thinking, "I can have that extra scoop of chocolate ice cream for dessert because I have lost a lot of weight and I am feeling really good". Just because you have lost weight it does not mean that extra calories do not add up anymore.

It is important to treat yourself from time to time, but it is also important to recognise when extra treats are creeping into your diet too often. By keeping a food diary (or just listing the extras you are having on a notepad) you can identify how frequently you are treating yourself. You should consume no more than 2-3 treats per week, and whenever you consume a treat limit yourself to a 200 Calorie portion.

8. Be Organised

It is hard to manage your weight when the rest of your life is in chaos. Leave plenty of time for relaxation, sleeping, shopping for healthy foods, preparing healthy meals and exercising.

9. Maintain your Self Esteem

Maintain a healthy level of self esteem - do not link how you feel about yourself to your weight. Be happy with you weight and proud of the weight loss that you have achieved.

10. Do Not Use Food to Stabilise Your Moods

If you are feeling stressed or upset, find a non-food related way of calming yourself - go for a walk, take a bath or call a friend.

Lastly, do not forget that weight maintenance can be just as challenging as weight loss (if not more so in the first two years). But it gets easier with time, and by following our advice you will be well on your way to success.

Strategies for Maintaining Weight Loss

Losing weight is difficult enough. But dieters are also faced with the fact that odds are stacked against them for long-term success. Researchers estimate that only about 20 percent of dieters maintain weight loss after a diet. Are you going to be one of them?

How to Maintain Weight Loss After a Diet

To increase your chances of weight maintenance after a diet, plan for a transitional phase after you reach your goal weight. During this time, make slow adjustments to your lifestyle and watch the effects on the scale. Abrupt changes are likely to cause weight regain.

This transitional phase is also a good time to identify the eating habits and exercise patterns that you learned while dieting so that you can maintain for the long term. If you turn healthy diet habits into healthy lifestyle habits, you're likely to prevent weight regain.

The 10 habits below will help you to move from the dieting phase, through the transitional phase and finally into the maintenance phase, where your weight remains stable. To improve your chances of permanent weight-loss success, try to incorporate these 10 habits into your lifestyle as you move through all phases of the dieting journey.

1. Moderate weight loss works best.

Physicians recommend that dieters lose no more than one to two pounds per week. This conservative approach helps patients avoid health risks associated with drastic weight loss. It also allows the dieter to learn new eating habits that will protect their weight loss in the long run. Portion control, healthy snacking, regular exercise, and reading nutritional labels are key skills that you'll master if you choose the slower approach to weight loss.

2. Make a slow transition out of the dieting stage.

Once you reach your goal weight, the worst thing you can do is to resume your old eating habits. Remember that those are the eating habits that caused the weight gain in the first place. It is reasonable to gradually increase caloric intake, but experts generally suggest adding only 200 calories per week until your weight stabilizes.

3. Stay connected to your sources of support.

The same people who supported you in the dieting process will help you maintain your weight loss. They are in the best position to respect the magnitude of your accomplishment and give you a gentle reminder if you lose track of your success. Communicate with them and give them permission to offer respectful guidance if needed.

4. Continue to challenge yourself with new goals.

Now that you've mastered one of the toughest challenges you'll ever face, stay on your toes by setting a new goal. It doesn't have to be related to weight loss. Achieving both short-term and long-term goals will help you keep your confidence level high.

5. Stay educated.

Take healthy-cooking classes, go to health seminars and participate in fitness fairs. Surround yourself with reminders of what living a healthy life really means. You may also want to stay involved online.

6. Become a mentor.

One of the best ways to stay educated is to teach your weight-loss skills to a newbie. By becoming a mentor, you'll be required to stay on top of new research and trends.

7. Exercise.

Research into permanent weight loss reveals that exercise is one of the best predictors of long-term success. Thirty to 60 minutes of moderate exercise every day will keep both your body and mind healthy.

8. Eat breakfast.

Studies have also found that people who eat breakfast are more successful at keeping the pounds at bay. Make sure that your breakfast includes whole grains and a lean source of protein.

9. Weigh yourself.

Keep a scale in your bathroom and use it once a week. Studies show that checking your weight on a regular basis is a practice shared by people who successfully keep their weight off.

10. Keep regular appointments with your healthcare team.

Your healthcare provider or registered dietician will be able to measure your body fat percentage or evaluate your BMI to make sure that your numbers stay healthy.

They will also be able to address health issues that arise when your body shape changes. Outside of the office, you can track your own progress by entering your measurements into an easy-to-use calculator like the one below.

<u>The strategies that encourage weight loss also play an important role in maintenance</u>:

Support systems used effectively during weight loss can contribute to weight maintenance. According to the National Weight Control Registry, 55% of registry participants used some type of program to achieve their weight loss.

Physical activity plays a vital and essential role in maintaining weight loss. Studies show that even exercise that is not rigorous, such as walking and using stairs, has a positive effect. Activity that uses 1,500 to 2,000 calories per week is recommended for maintaining weight loss. Adults should try to get at least 40 minutes of moderate to vigorous level physical activity at least 3 to 4 times per week.

Diet and exercise are vital strategies for losing and maintaining weight. Ninety-four percent of the registrants in the National Weight Control Registry increased their physical activity.

Once the desired weight has been reached, the gradual addition of about 200 calories of healthy, low-fat food to daily intake may be attempted for one week to see if weight loss continues. If weight loss does continue, additional calories of healthy foods may be added to the daily diet until the right balance of calories to maintain the desired weight has been determined. It may take some time and record keeping to determine how adjusting food intake and exercise levels affect weight. A nutritionist can help with this.

Continuing to use behavioral strategies is necessary to maintaining weight. Be aware of eating as a response to stress. Also, use exercise, activity, or meditation to cope instead of eating.

A temporary return to old habits does not mean failure. Paying attention to dietary choices and exercise can help maintain weight loss. Identifying situations, such as negative moods and interpersonal difficulties, and using alternative methods of coping with such situations rather than eating can prevent returning to old habits.

CONCLUSION

The DASH diet, which does not include sodium reduction or weight loss, had significant blood-pressure-lowering effects in virtually all subgroups. These effects were particularly striking in African Americans and in those with stage 1 hypertension. This intervention adds to our current nonpharmacologic approaches to control high blood pressure. The DASH diet may be an effective strategy for preventing and treating hypertension in a broad cross-section of the population, including those at high risk for hypertension and its complications.